Introducing Research and Evidence-Based Practice for Nursing and Healthcare Professionals

Second edition

Jeremy Jolley

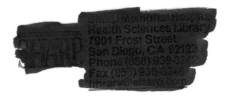

PEARSON

Harlow, England • London • New York • Boston • San Francisco • Toronto • Sydney • Auckland • Singapore • Hong Kong
Tokyo • Seoul • Taipei • New Delhi • Cape Town • São Paulo • Mexico City • Madrid • Amsterdam • Munich • Paris • Milan

Pearson Education Limited
Edinburgh Gate
Harlow
Essex CM20 2JE
England

and Associated Companies throughout the world

Visit us on the World Wide Web at:
www.pearson.com/uk

First published 2010
This edition published 2013

ISBN 978-0-273-76885-2

British Library Cataloguing-in-Publication Data
A catalogue record for this book is available from the British Library

Library of Congress Cataloging-in-Publication Data
A catalog record for this book is available from the Library of Congress

10 9 8 7 6 5 4 3 2 1
16 15 14 13 12

Typeset in 10.25/14pt Interstate Light by 35
Printed and bound in Malaysia (CTP-PJB)

To Susan, Alice and Catherine

Contents

Preface

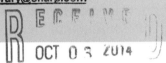
This book has been written for those who are new to research and who may struggle to understand what it is all about. Of course, there are already lots of books on research. There are big books, complicated books, books that try to summarise the whole subject of research. Many of these books are tedious, stuffy and often incomprehensible to those new to the subject. This book is different: it deals only with the important aspects of healthcare research, what practitioners need to know for research to begin to make real sense. This book isn't stuffy. Real research is exciting; it is imagining something new; it is dealing with real-life questions and finding answers; it is making healthcare better for real patients and real practitioners.

The subject that is research can sometimes look complex and perplexing; it can make people feel unintelligent and lost. This book aims to put that right, to show the reader that research can be understood, that research is at its core really simple and genuinely useful. All healthcare practitioners are clever people and no one gets as far as reading a book like this without possessing real vigour and enthusiasm for the subject they have chosen to study and to practise. We should all believe in ourselves; healthcare practice is our responsibility and we need to understand research and evidence-based practice to ensure that healthcare continues to grow and to develop.

Nurses and healthcare practitioners often don't get the opportunity to experience research, to work on a real research project. This lack of a research-practice element to our studies makes it hard for us to understand what research is all about. We all learn by seeing and doing, and a lack of research practice makes it hard for us to understand research.

Healthcare practice, including medicine, exists as a particularly broad range of disciplines and, as a result of this, employs almost every kind of research strategy that exists. Healthcare practice, from nursing to physiotherapy to medicine, employs both quantitative and qualitative approaches to research. As such, we see the use of everything from surveys to experiments to approaches that seek one person's understanding of another at the deepest psychological and emotional level. The richness and diversity of research in healthcare practice leaves other occupational groups standing, but it also means that it is much more difficult for healthcare practitioners to get to grips with research. Let us be perfectly clear: there is a lot to healthcare research. It is sad that so very few existing texts try to help the learning practitioner through this maze. This book is different: it aims to provide just such guidance, to hold the reader's hand through the journey of discovery. The book does this, while consistently valuing the subject matter, its central importance to healthcare, the intelligence of each and every practitioner and the potential each of us carries within us to produce real advances in patient care.

This second edition has enabled a welcome opportunity to add two chapters on qualitative research. Qualitative articles are usually written in accessible English and the common use of the first person has the effect of making them seem friendly. The research itself often addresses the more human and emotive side of healthcare, which many students find interesting. However, anyone who has taken more than a glance at qualitative research will appreciate that it has a sting in its tail. For just beneath the surface, qualitative research gets seriously complex. Those who have turned their back on statistics and double-blind trials find themselves mixed up instead in nineteenth-century philosophy and wordy sociological constructs. The experience is like going for a walk on a pleasant summer's day only to fall into a muddy hole in the ground, wondering how on earth one came to such a place.

Fear not, for in the spirit of the first edition, this text will lead the reader gently through the quagmire of convoluted terminology and constructs that is qualitative research. Just like quantitative research, its qualitative partner is actually really, really, simple. In fact, it is possible to write down how we undertake qualitative research (how it is done) on one side of a sheet of paper (I've done it, here). Of course, we shall look at qualitative research pragmatically, because healthcare practitioners are pragmatic people, interested in doing and understanding research, not for its own sake but rather to help us make things better for patients and clients.

Acknowledgements

We are grateful to the following for permission to reproduce copyright material:

Figures

Figure 2.1 from www.ebscohost.com, (c) EBSCO Publishing, Inc., 2009. All rights reserved; Figures 2.2, 2.3 from EBSCO, (c) EBSCO Publishing, Inc., 2009. All rights reserved; Figure 3.1 Author's own image – taken in the early 1920s at the now closed Victoria Children's Hospital (Hull). The image was taken by a nurse who died a few years ago; Figure 5.1 from Wong's *Essentials of Pediatric Nursing*, 7th ed, Mosby (Hockenberry, M.J., Wilson D., Winkelstein, M.L. 2005) p.1259

In some instances we have been unable to trace the owners of copyright material, and we would appreciate any information that would enable us to do so.

Chapter 1
Research is simple

CHAPTER OBJECTIVES

The objectives for this chapter are to:

- Suggest that research *is* relevant to healthcare practice
- Show that research can be interesting and even fun
- Argue that, although research looks complex, it is in fact readily understandable and you know a lot of it already.

Chapter outline

People often find it difficult to understand the real meaning of the terms 'research' and 'evidence-based practice'. This chapter aims to make it possible for anyone to understand what these terms mean and why they are relevant to healthcare. In short, this chapter will help you make sense of what can sometimes seem a complex area of study. Research can seem to be complex, but this chapter will show you that research is really very simple. Indeed, this chapter will convince you that you already know about research.

What is research?

You are probably reading this because you have been asked to study research or evidence-based practice. Perhaps you have been asked to write your first research proposal. Research can seem complex, but it is actually little more than what you already do and what you already know. Fundamentally, research is simple and this book aims to keep it that way.

Research is relevant to you and it is relevant to healthcare practice. In fact, research and practice are inseparable. Practice needs to be questioning, it needs to seek to find better ways to help people; practice needs research. Indeed, research is similar to the questioning and investigative stance that clinical practitioners use all of the time. Think about it: when you first see a patient or client, you will want to talk with them, watch them and ask them questions. Your assessment of the patient isn't haphazard or random; it is organised, it is systematic. This systematic approach to the gathering of information is not only similar to research – it is what *defines* research. Research is not just any old haphazard collection of data; research is organised, thought-through and systematised – exactly like your assessment of a new patient. Furthermore, in your own practice you will use skills that are identical to the skills used in research. You will, for example, try to collect data that are rich enough (sufficient enough) for your purpose, and you will use data collection methods that are purposeful and thought-through – just as in a research project. When you see a new patient, you use a face-to-face interview; you do not give them a questionnaire or get them involved in a focus group. So it is with research: research uses the most appropriate means of data collection, and that may be and often is exactly the technique you use when assessing a new patient.

Healthcare students do sometimes become confused about research. They find that they are unsure about what research is. Now we know why they are confused. Research is what practice is, and practice is what research is. No wonder students are confused – they are looking for something new to study

New words

Data (Datum) Values or factual information collected during research. Note that 'data' is plural, so that a researcher might say 'these data are interesting'. The singular form is 'datum'.

when in fact they have been living and breathing it since the first day of their course. You already know about research; it is in every fibre of your enquiring mind and you can use it to contribute to nursing and make things better.

Let us be clear: you are studying research because you have a lively and intelligent mind; in fact, you have already acquired so much knowledge of research that you will not find your present studies difficult. Indeed, you already know most of the important principles of research.

You may be concerned that you are not very good at mathematics; well, that's no problem. Researchers need only to use computer applications that deal with numbers, as a word processor deals with words. Don't worry if you are not good with numbers. Many researchers are not good with numbers either.

Let's start by defining research. Have a look at the definitions listed in Table 1.1.

Table 1.1 Definitions of research

Scientific method	The scientific method is a sort of philosophical underpinning for everything we call science. It is very similar to the nursing process in that it is systematic and objective. It goes something like this:
	1. The hunch (a gut feeling about a possible enquiry)
	2. Literature review to find out what is already known
	3. Problem identification
	4. The hypothesis
	5. Plan for research
	6. Data collection
	7. Data analysis
	8. Discussion of results/evaluation
Research	Research is any enquiry that is systematic in its approach and that seeks to ensure that the results of the enquiry cannot be criticised on the grounds of poor technique
Evidence-based practice	Evidence-based practice is said to exist where there is a clear attempt to base clinical practice upon known evidence. Research evidence is usually the best form of evidence, but sometimes other forms of evidence are used

Figure 1.1 shows the relationship between three important concepts. The purpose of science and of research is to produce practice that is based on evidence; that is, practice that is understood and is known to be effective.

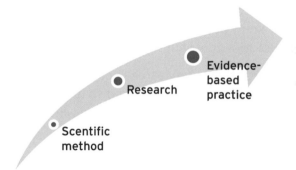

Figure 1.1 Relationship between three important concepts in nursing.

New words

Robust A word that means 'solid' or 'unshakable' and that is applied to research studies that are difficult to criticise. Qualitative studies often use the word 'trustworthy' instead.

Quantitative research This is research that we most clearly associate with traditional science. Quantitative research usually deals with numbers rather than text and, as the term suggests, deals with the 'quantity' of something. For example, we might measure patients' anxiety by asking them to allocate a number from 1 to 5 to indicate how anxious they are.

Qualitative research This is research that deals mostly with language or text. As the name suggests, it is concerned with the quality of something. For example, we might interview patients about their anxiety. This would allow patients to talk about their lived experience of anxiety, what that experience meant to them and how it affected their daily lives.

So, what *is* research? All research is nothing more than systematic enquiry. Quantitative research is an endeavour to discover new information, in a manner that is structured, systematic and objective, while using techniques (methodologies) that are robust. Qualitative research is also systematic (it has a defined method or 'plan') but allows for the interpretation of data in a manner that may be subjective but which is open to audit. All researchers want to produce research of good quality (research that is robust or trustworthy). If the methodology is questionable, so will be the results. The definition of research given here applies to all research, from that which takes place in laboratories to that which focuses on human experiences. All research is just a systematic enquiry.

The 'salt bath' and poor methodology

Healthcare practitioners are good at using sound principles for the collection of data. However, occasionally those sound principles have not been well applied. The history of the salt bath is interesting because it warns us to be on our guard against poor methodologies.

Through most of the twentieth century, salt baths were used to help heal wounds. Patients could often be found relaxing in baths to which had been added a variable amount of table salt (Austin 1988). It had long been argued that salt baths were more or less essential for wound healing to take place.

Now, let us prove that salt baths do work. Let's do an experiment. The next time you cut your finger, put it into a cup of water with salt in it (it doesn't matter how much salt). Do this three times a day (because 'three times a day' sounds very therapeutic). Your finger will get better. So, salt baths work; we have proved it.

Of course, you will have seen that our methodology is less than robust. The chances are that your finger would have got better without the salt-water treatment. Wounds have a tendency to get better all on their own. The problem here is that we did not set up a control. If we had tested, say, 50 cut fingers given no treatment and 50 cut fingers given a saline bath, then we would find that being dipped in saline three times a day made no difference whatsoever to the healing rate or the incidence of successful healing.

However, before we criticise practitioners in the past for their lack of research (see Walsh and Ford 1989), we should bear in mind that healthcare is a big discipline containing a great deal of expertise. We are all human and it is difficult to question practices that are long established and widely accepted. When you next go to work, take a look at what you find yourself doing and ask 'What exactly is the evidence that this works?'

Research – a two-headed beast

It will probably not surprise you that there is more than one form of research. You are probably aware that a survey, for example, is not the same thing as an experiment. Research does come in several different forms. For the moment, however, it would be useful to introduce the two main research variants. Arguably, every research study will fit into one or other of these two variants:

- *Quantitative research*: this deals in quantities of things. The data from quantitative studies exist usually in the form of numbers, which can then be quantified (added up) and subjected to statistical analysis. Quantitative research is often used to 'demonstrate' the truth in a hypothesis; that is, to demonstrate that something we think is true, is actually true.

- *Qualitative research*: this deals in the quality of things. However, this definition is not very helpful. In practice, this category of research deals in data that exist as words and concepts rather than as numbers. Qualitative research is often used to 'explore' human experience, especially where the researcher simply doesn't know enough about that experience even to know what questions to ask, so prompts such as 'Tell me about your experience of [whatever]' are often used.

These two categories almost represent fields of research, with researchers often spending their whole career in one field or the other. This can lead to researchers valuing one approach over the other. However, it is possible to make use of both quantitative and qualitative forms of research and even of mixing the two approaches together within the same study (Canning *et al.* 2007). In any case, healthcare practice needs both forms of research and we should try to value what each can provide. We may need to 'test something out' – we have an idea about improving practice and we want to see if it works. Often, quantitative research works best for this. However, we also need to know how what we do is 'experienced' by patients and clients. Such a question is often best dealt with using qualitative research. In time, the results from qualitative research and our better understanding of what patients and clients experience will lead us to examine specific aspects of that experience and this can often be done using quantitative research designs. In this way, both

Example from the literature and research

Meyers *et al.* (2004) used a quantitative approach to study the experience of family members being present during invasive procedures and resuscitation. It was found that family members were positive about their experience and considered being present to be their right. There was found to be no evidence of psychological trauma to family members who stayed with their loved one during resuscitation. The study found that nurses and senior doctors tended to be in favour of family members being present with the patient, but junior doctors tended to be less happy. Perhaps nurses and senior doctors are more confident about the care they provide during invasive procedures and resuscitation than are junior doctors and are thus more willing to be watched at a time when nursing and medical skills are critical to the patient's survival.

Example from the literature and research

Wigert *et al.* (2006) conducted a qualitative study into mothers' experience of their newborn child being in intensive care. Using interviews with mothers, it was found that the mother often felt excluded from the social environment of the unit and that this then had a negative effect on her maternal feelings toward her own baby. The implications of this study are that staff should make mothers feel welcome and should help mothers to feel valued and useful. This will not only make mothers feel better about themselves but will also enable them to develop a normal and warm relationship with their child.

quantitative and qualitative approaches to research are not only useful, but complement each other.

You already know about research

Research is essentially a simple activity. However, research often looks complex and research studies can be quite large. Research is simple but it possesses its own language, which can take time to learn. Research uses a range of techniques to ensure that the resulting data are what they are meant to be and not biased or unreliable. These techniques can look complex at first, but they are not complex. Then there are those numbers; statistical analyses can look very complex. However, appearances are deceptive and the most advanced and apparently complex statistic will always be simple and intuitive at its core. Furthermore, it is the principles of research that you should learn now. For example, by the end of this book you will understand the rationale for using inferential statistics, but you will not need to learn how to calculate every single statistical procedure. With these principles in your pocket, you will know all you need to know about research and, indeed, you will be ready to use research in your own area of clinical practice.

New words

Bias The unwanted inclusion of extraneous factors that influence the results of a study.

Reliability The degree to which further implementation of a study will yield the same results.

Research is systematic enquiry and is something with which you are already very familiar. Say that you are looking for material for an essay on the management of post-surgery pain. You go to the library and you go to the section on pain management and then perhaps to the section on surgery. You might do an electronic literature search using the keywords 'surgery' and 'pain'. Finally, you might go and have a word with one of the faculty staff members who has done some work in this area. That's good. You have undertaken a search, but not just any old search: your search has been goal-orientated and systematic. You didn't look in the history of art section of the library; nor did you ask that student who keeps failing her essay for help. You thought about it, not wanting to waste your time. You wanted to be focused, to be clear about what you were looking for. There is no material difference between this and research.

Perhaps you think that research is more complex because it often includes experiments, difficult language and lots of numbers. Not at all; in fact, you used a library – and lots of people can't do that. You used an electronic search engine – most people can't do that. Importantly, you used a goal-orientated and systematic approach – hardly anyone can do that (just watch MPs in the House of Commons trying to decide something). The fact is, you are brilliant, a real achiever, a star. Seriously, you are a very clever person. In fact, you already do research and what there is left to learn will come easily and intuitively.

What has research to do with healthcare practice?

Students at the beginning of their programme of study are often surprised to discover that they are expected to learn about research. When asked why they wish to be nurses, physiotherapists or theatre technicians, many interviewees will say that they want to make a difference to peoples' lives by doing something to help in times of illness or distress. Interviewees will often indicate that they are practical people with a gift for getting on with others and that they want to do a socially useful job. It would be unusual in the extreme to come across a candidate who wanted to enter healthcare practice because of a desire to research or to spend their time in academia.

The fact that newcomers to the profession are sometimes surprised to learn even that there is such a thing as non-medical healthcare research probably has something to do with the image of research and the image of nursing and paramedical healthcare disciplines. When you have a moment, use your computer to search for images of research. You will find pictures of men and women in white coats peering into microscopes, rows of test tubes in laboratories and complex flow diagrams covered with tiny writing. Now look for images of nurses (for example). You will find pictures of uniformed men and women dealing with sick people in hospital. These images will be of nurses doing clinical things such as taking blood pressure readings and helping people to walk (while invariably smiling). The words 'nursing' and 'research' seem to have little in common. Of course, it just takes a moment's reflection to realise that these are very simplistic depictions of both research and nursing, but in a way that's precisely the point: there is more to both nursing and research than there might at first appear to be. Research, for example, does not always use expensive equipment in hi-tech laboratories. Sometimes, researchers will collect information using a method based on something we can all do – speaking to another person and listening carefully to what they say in response. Equally, the variety and complexity of nursing are not easily or accurately represented by the familiar stereotypes of paper caps, crisp uniforms and hospital beds.

Practice and research – the same motivation

Why do you turn up for work in the morning? Initially, practitioners are often motivated by a desire to help and support other people in practical ways (Rognstad and Aasland 2007); this is probably true of you. We need to look no further than this to find a major source of motivation for quite a lot of research. Most of the research that you will read about in journals and textbooks will have been undertaken by practitioners. Some of these practitioners will have done the research while working in a clinical role, while some research will have been carried out by people working as teachers and researchers in university departments; however, nearly all of it will have been done by people with a professional qualification. People don't stop being clinical practitioners when they become researchers; the motivation that led them to their profession is the same motivation that leads them to undertake and publish research projects. You can see this by turning to a journal and looking at the titles of the articles that are published there to get a sense of what they are about. The subjects that are being investigated will often relate to everyday clinical problems and concerns.

Why knowledge can't simply be passed on from one person to another

Clinical practitioners, in their everyday work, try to help people to solve problems related to their health. Sometimes problems are entirely unique to one particular individual, while at other times they fall into patterns. For example, it's very common for patients to experience pain in various circumstances, and the practitioner will want to relieve this if they can; and although each person's pain is unique in the sense that they are the only person who can feel it, experienced practitioners learn that peoples' stories of pain tend to have common features, not least of which is that pain is generally considered to be unpleasant. As practitioners build up a bank of experience, they may try a number of different ways of addressing these problems, some of which seem to work at least some of the time, while others are rather less useful. On occasion they may resort to traditional approaches that they have learned from others and, again, they may have variable rates of success as they use these methods. One of the problems of working on your own or in a small team is that you can build up what we might call 'customary' ways of working. Certain habits of practice develop. The problem is that it can be very difficult for an individual practitioner or a small group of practitioners working together on a ward to get an objective sense of the effectiveness of what they are doing.

Here is an account by a lecturer in nursing, looking back at his early experience as a student nurse:

> One of my first experiences as a student nurse was to be shown a traditional way of caring for a patient with a pressure sore. The patient was a man with advanced multiple sclerosis, and he had a sore the size of a 10p coin on his bottom. The ward sister showed me how to roll the patient on to his side, and then used a brush to apply beaten egg white to the sore. Next, she used a plastic tube to blow oxygen on to the egg white to dry it.

> I was a bit surprised at this treatment and asked the sister what benefit it was. She explained that pressure sores occurred when tissue was poorly nourished and badly oxygenated. Thus, there was clearly a logic to what she was doing, though looking back I suspect that the simple act of turning the patient on to his side for a while was of more use than the egg white and oxygen.

In recent years, nurse researchers have investigated many traditional treatments of this kind and found that they simply don't work (Helberg *et al.* 2006). Research is a way of testing our practice and finding out which approaches are most effective. This is sometimes known as clinical effectiveness.

There is a lot of knowledge out there and practitioners know how to do a lot of things. You can, for example, pick up a copy of the current *European Resuscitation Council Guidelines* (Baskett and Zideman 2005), read them and know what to do when someone needs to be resuscitated. In the same way, there exists a plethora of textbooks that the enquiring practitioner can use to guide practice. So, why is there a need for research? Why not wait until all the research becomes incorporated into the textbooks and then just read the textbooks?

If you wait for this to happen, you are not participating in your profession. It's like waiting for someone to cook your dinner and then waiting for someone else to do the washing up. You are just sitting on the couch getting fat. Your healthcare discipline is *your* discipline: it isn't run for you, you are running it. There isn't anyone to do the washing up – you have to do it. If you want to eat, you have to cook your own dinner. Your chosen healthcare discipline belongs to you. As a clinical practitioner, you have a responsibility to make things better, to take things forward, to improve the service that is offered to patients. What we know now is not good enough; it can never be good enough because it can be even better. Your job is to make it better, and research is the key way to make that happen. It is in this way that the healthcare disciplines are regarded as professions. If it were just a job, you could indeed wait for someone to tell you what to do. What you do is not just a job: you have a responsibility not only to your patients and not only to one particular shift and to your hospital or team but also to your profession. It is not good enough that you provide expert care only to your patient; you must also provide expert care, research and leadership to the whole profession.

Patients and others who depend on us should be certain that 'their' healthcare practitioner is doing more than obeying orders or following the guidelines found in textbooks. From the most junior student to the consultant, people need to be aware of research and aware of the gaps in research where we are still ignorant of how best to help patients. However, even this is not enough: every practitioner should be capable of addressing the gaps in our knowledge and of seeking out ways to increase our understanding, so that practitioners everywhere are better able to provide the best care that is possible.

A practice discipline

Your discipline is a practice discipline; it has no purpose beyond its practice. For this reason, healthcare research is almost wholly inductive; that is, it seeks to answer questions about practice. Most healthcare disciplines do not have a well-defined concept base; there are no real theories of nursing or occupational therapy as there are theoretical perspectives in psychology, such as Freudian theory and behaviourism. Clinical research does not, on the whole, seek to produce either theory or pure knowledge, as do disciplines such as psychology and sociology. Practice disciplines do not seek to produce either knowledge or theory for its own sake; rather, they seek to be able to do more and to be more effective.

New words

Theory A mature set of interrelated ideas supported by at least some evidence. In time, even well-developed theory may be shown to be wrong.

Inductive research Research raised from questions about practice rather than from theory. Inductive research can be used to generate new theory, but it usually exists to answer gaps in our knowledge.

Deductive research Research that is derived from theory. This is unusual in nursing but more common in psychology, where, for example, one might speak of 'psychoanalytical research' (research that stems from psychoanalytical theory).

There is a study element to research. However, there is a study element to the life of every professional person. Learning is a life-long process in any profession. The student who thinks that 3 years of study will set them up for a lifetime of practice is misguided. So, yes, there is a study element to research. One has to learn how to find research and then how to read it, interpret it, practise it and implement research into practice. Get used to the idea, for it is common to professional life. For a full professional life, there must be study and practice. Research is almost always directed at questions of practice and is purposed to improve the work of all practitioners for the benefit of the patient.

Where is research?

Research can sometimes seem invisible, but it is present and is eminently practical in nature. When you first started in clinical practice, you probably found it all a little confusing. You had to find the ward, then the ward office. Later on, you struggled to find the nasogastric tubes and the dermatology department. For a while, it was confusing. Eventually, however, you worked out where everything was and you began to feel at home in your clinical environment.

Perhaps you have come to feel a sense of mastery over it all and you can now be found telling more junior students what to do and where to go to find things. However, research may be something that you have never really managed to make much sense of. After all, where is it? Where is the research department? Ages ago, you worked out what dermatology is, but what is research? Surely any self-respecting thing ought at least to be visible? So it is that you may have relegated research to the weird and ephemeral, like theory and philosophy. After all, if research was real, you would see the staff practising it and talking about it; it would have become part of what you do.

The truth is that, for many practitioners, research is something other people do; for many practitioners, research is indeed weird and ephemeral. You will have asked yourself how this could be. More importantly, you will have asked why you are being asked to study research when there are lots of other, more practical, things that you could be learning. The fact is that your discipline is developing. What you see around you is not what your discipline was 30 years ago and it is not what it will be in 30 years' time. The non-medical disciplines are in the process of developing into fully fledged professions. They have come a long way but there is still a distance to be travelled. So it is that your pro-gramme of study is preparing you not for the past, and not even for today, but for your practice tomorrow.

Healthcare cannot afford to stand still. It must always be searching for better ways of caring for people and it should never be satisfied with the ways things are now. So, your course should not fit exactly with what you see others doing in practice. You are the future of your profession and you are learning to prac-tise in the future. When you first started, you probably wanted to be just like the others in your discipline – you wanted to be an accepted member of the team, to know the routine and to look and feel like a professional. That is as it should be, but sooner or later you will have to learn how to be yourself, to be your own sort of practitioner and to imprint yourself on the future of your dis-cipline. You have seen the staff and tried to be like them. However, the time will come when you will have to create the future from your unique skills and your enthusiasm to make things better. Research is about moving things forward, rather than learning what other people already know.

Let us leave your own discipline for a moment and look at the disciplines of psychology and medicine; let's see if we can find research there. Psychology is split broadly into two career pathways: clinical psychology and academic psychology. Most psychology research is conducted by academic psychologists working in universities. So psychology students have no difficulty working out where to find research: as they go through their programme of study, research will be all around them.

So where is research in medicine? You know that there is research in medicine. You will have heard about the struggle to cure diseases for which treatment is still largely ineffective. You will have heard of research that led to the development of vaccines for such diseases as smallpox and poliomyelitis, which once wrought death and grief on a massive scale. If you work in a large teaching hospital you will even find that there are medical research departments. Your hospital might have a cardiac research department, for example. However, smaller hospitals often lack these research departments, so why is this? Most medical research takes place in universities. The larger teaching hospitals are staffed by the very same medical people who work in the universities and so you see research taking place there. However, in the non-teaching hospitals, the medical staff do not tend to have academic posts and so less research is carried out. It is different for the medical staff in smaller hospitals; for them, research is largely something other people do. However, all doctors take seriously their responsibility to ensure that their practice is grounded in current research.

So medicine is not perfect; but remember that you are learning to work in the future, not the present. The influence of research is growing very quickly. Even today, there are many practitioners for whom research is a central part of their working lives. Research is all around them and they live and breathe research every day. Suggest to any of these people that research is dry, academic and hard to define and they will look at you as if you have come from another planet. If they should have sufficient patience with you, they will pause and explain that research is anything but dry and academic. They will tell you that research is eminently practical; it is logically construed and orientated to finding answers to the everyday problems of clinical practice. Ask them to show you a researcher and you will be shown someone with their sleeves rolled up, doing work that could not be regarded as anything other than practical and pragmatic. If you thought that research was dry and academic, or ill-defined and nebulous, you were wrong.

So research is a very practical craft. It is, in fact, at the practical end of practice; it is more practical than much of the day-to-day work that goes on in clinical areas. So you asked your professor to show you a researcher and you were shown a real person doing seriously practical work. You asked the researcher what was involved in the work and what was the goal of it and you received a brief and plain reply. The work of the researcher is eminently practical.

The role of research in clinical practice

Let's think of an imaginary example of the role research plays in everyday practice:

> *Joe is a lively 9-year-old who loves to play football in his school team. One day he jumps to head a ball but accidentally collides with the goal post and cuts his head. The cut is about 2cm long and there is blood all over the place. Joe's parents take him to the accident and emergency department of the local hospital. A nurse makes an initial assessment. The nurse asks Joe how he cut his head and asks his parents whether he lost consciousness. She then uses glue to stick the edges of the wound together before sending Joe and his parents home.*

This is a brief description of a simple event. Things like this happen every day and will be very familiar to anyone with accident and emergency experience. However, you may be surprised to learn just how much of the interaction is shaped by the findings of research.

Children can have a serious and life-threatening head injury without having a fractured skull and with very little bruising. However, practitioners know how to determine whether a child is likely to have a minor or a serious head injury; they consider prognostic indicators such as those identified by Kieslich *et al.* (2001). If practitioners based their practice on experience alone, then it would take them hundreds of years to learn what prognostic indicators could be used effectively.

Dealing with Joe's wound may be both frightening and painful. The practitioner may decide to use distraction to help Joe deal effectively with the investigation and treatment of his wound. However, the practitioner will want to use a form of distraction that is known to be reliable and so he or she chooses to base this practice on research such as that by Windich-Biermeier *et al.* (2007). This study demonstrates that, when performed properly, distraction can be a valuable tool in helping children cope with fearful and painful procedures.

The glue that the practitioner uses to close Joe's wound will have been chosen for its effectiveness. All glues sting a little, but research has demonstrated which glues are maximally effective while causing the least discomfort to children (Charters 2000).

As you watch this practitioner in action, you might be forgiven for thinking that he or she is simply doing what is common sense or perhaps what he or she has been trained to do. You look at the practitioner, quietly and competently helping Joe; you do not see the research. However, in this simple scenario, research is everywhere. The practitioner's actions are guided at almost every step by research.

This little example has begun to illustrate some of the reasons for our involvement in research and to show why practitioners are expected to learn about research and to apply the findings in their practice when they become qualified. We have already made the point that people are often surprised by the extent and importance of clinical research because they imagine, quite wrongly, that practice and research are two entirely different things.

Who does research today?

Just as research itself can be hidden from the world of practice, so too can be the people who carry out research. Most nursing research, for example, is probably undertaken by nurses who work in universities. However, we have noted that all healthcare research has a practice focus and the studies that take place tend to involve practice areas, patients, clients and professional staff.

Research tends to be expensive. People's time costs money and research projects can take a long time to complete. The agencies providing research funding need to make sure that their funds are used wisely – so funding tends to go to research teams that have a known history of producing good research. These research teams are likely to be based in one or more universities. However, those who fund research will usually want to see evidence of collaboration with the practice setting and, because of this, there are opportunities for practice staff to become involved in research – so most good research is managed by university staff in close collaboration with clinical staff. There are important exceptions to this, but it is still the case that the universities do and will continue to play a central role in the conduct of research studies.

As a student, you stand with one foot in the university and one foot in practice. You will probably see your future in practice and you look forward to the day when you will have both of your feet in the practice setting. It may be wise, however, to consider maintaining your links with your university. Research is as much a part of practice as medical research is part of medicine. This is a difficult but important idea to accept, especially for the student who may see their passage through the university as transient and self-limiting. In fact, you have embarked on a lifelong-learning profession and, as such, your relationship with the university should not end when you graduate. You will never stop having ideas about how practice could be improved, and it is sometimes good to share those ideas with university staff so that your discipline can be developed to improve the care provided to patients and clients. This is rightly a bilateral relationship. Practitioners know where they are frustrated by an inability to provide the patient or client with what is needed. University staff have the research expertise to develop a study that could move our knowledge forward. This collaboration of equal partners is an effective model for the building of research projects for the improvement of nursing care.

The message is clear: when you leave university, don't leave. If you have left university, go back. This does not mean that you should go back to undertake another course of study but that you should go back to maintain effective links with academic staff. In this way, ideas are shared, projects are started, and the boundaries of practice and of science are pushed back – by people like you.

Try this: Go to the Dean of your faculty or search out one of the professors – go on, corner them! Ask them for a list of ongoing research taking place within the faculty. List those research projects in the space provided below. You may be surprised just how much research activity is going on all around you.

(1) _____   (10) _____

(2) _____   (11) _____

(3) _____   (12) _____

(4) _____   (13) _____

(5) _____   (14) _____

(6) _____   (15) _____

(7) _____   (16) _____

(8) _____   (17) _____

(9) _____   (18) _____

Now do one last thing: choose one of the studies taking place in your faculty, from the list you made above – select something that looks interesting. Go and see the person in charge of this project and ask them to tell you about their project. Get the following details about their study:

- The title

- The duration of the project

- What the study aims to achieve

- How the study relates to practice.

So, we have noted that most research is undertaken within universities but in close collaboration with clinical staff. It is unfortunate that a lot of research is invisible to the casual observer, even to students. However, if you just ask, you will find that research is already everywhere.

Research: what's in it for me?

There are two main reasons why people become involved in research:

- To push forward the frontiers of science

- To push forward the frontiers of their career.

These two goals do not have to be in conflict. However, the acceptance of research in professional practice is sometimes limited by the belief that researchers are simply furthering their own career. Think about it, though: how many wealthy researchers do you know? No one ever made a fortune out of research. Furthermore, it is no bad thing to want to progress one's career. Take a look at the people you meet in your clinical area; some of them will be happy to do what they are doing now until they retire. That's good because good practice needs good experience. However, look around you again; in fact, go and search out those practitioners who have progressed their career and talk to them about it. Go and talk with your clinical manager or leader. Here are some questions you can ask them:

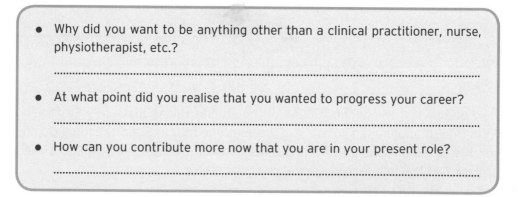

- Why did you want to be anything other than a clinical practitioner, nurse, physiotherapist, etc.?

  ....

- At what point did you realise that you wanted to progress your career?

  ....

- How can you contribute more now that you are in your present role?

  ....

Being involved in research is one way in which practitioners can contribute more. A ward or community nurse, for example, does a great job; it is the job to which you may rightly aspire. However, nurses are not static creatures but find that they are able to deliver more as they gain experience, skills and knowledge. When you qualify and begin to work as a ward or community nurse (for example), you will be doing a fantastic job. That job will be uniquely practical and intellectual, and it will be rewarding on many different levels. However, it won't be easy: you have chosen one of the most difficult programmes of study ever offered by universities, and you are looking forward to doing a job that will tax every fibre of your body, mind and soul. It is precisely this sense of endeavour, this willingness to do more than what is easy and comfortable, that will drive you on to do more and more with your career. Importantly, you will come to a point in your career when you can deliver expert patient care. It is at that point that you will want to begin to influence not only what you can do but what all nurses can do. At this point, you will want to make a difference not only to one or two patients but to many patients.

As a ward or community nurse, you will find yourself addressing this question: How can I ensure that this patient's pain is controlled more capably? Sooner or later, you will find yourself asking: How can nurses better manage patients' pain?

This will be your defining moment. Go back to the responses you wrote down in the box above. You will find that those you spoke to can express that defining moment and the difference it has made to their outlook and their career.

Being involved in research is one way that practitioners can make a difference on a scale that is wider than the day-to-day care of their patients. However, researchers do not need to work with patient care *or* research; they can, and they do, do both.

Being a researcher may not be on your priority list just now, but one day it may be. This is the way it is because you are intelligent enough to be doing one of the most demanding courses available. You are courageous enough to enter a profession that is well outside your comfort zone. You want to make things better for those who suffer. You are the stuff of progress, initiative and adventure. You could become a great researcher.

In the coming years you will be stamping your own mark on your profession and re-fashioning it to improve it and make it right for the years ahead. There can be no doubt that research will play a bigger part in your practice in the future, in your future. The migration of the healthcare disciplines to research and evidence-led professions is already under way. In the years to come, there will be no confusion about what clinical research is or where it can be found; it will be everywhere. This shouldn't be frightening because you already value exactly what research values – that is, practice, a clear, objective focus and a demand that your discipline should never rest on its laurels but should instead be constantly researching new ways to deliver better, more effective, care.

This chapter started by wondering where research could be found, and we thought that research must be both academic and irrelevant to the practice of healthcare. We have come to see that research will develop in the future as the healthcare professions develop. We have also seen that research is far from being dry and academic; rather, it is a practical endeavour, goaled to improve the care that practitioners are able to deliver. Research in healthcare is essential because the healthcare professions will never be content with what they know and what they can do. Your discipline, led as it will be, by you, will always strive to make things better.

Example from practice

What do you want to be doing in 5 years' time?

Just now you will be occupied with successfully completing your course. You will be looking forward to being a qualified practitioner. You may not have looked much further than this; after all, this is quite a big achievement. However, it can be useful to think about a longer-term vision. Take a few moments to jot down where you would like to be at the following points in your career:

- In 2 years' time, or when you first feel that you are expert at your first post-qualifying post
- In 5 years' time, when you will have lots of experience and may want to branch out and specialise
- When you have been in practice long enough that people look to you because of your experience and knowledge.

What kind of practitioner do you want to be?

Give this some thought and then tick just one of the following boxes:

- I want to be a proper nurse, physio, theatre practitioner, etc. to look like a member of my profession and be respected for my practice. I want to be like the other people who work in my area of practice and work as a member of a team, with them. ☐
- I want to work with other practitioners in my field and be good at what I do, but I also want to find my own mark and make my own unique contribution to my profession and to patient care. ☐

Which one is correct? That depends on you; both represent a significant achievement. However, there is an important distinction between the two answers. It is worth some thought. Pester the researchers in your faculty just one more time and ask them which box they would tick.

Concluding remarks

It is often thought that research is a dry and academic subject and one that is not at all suited to the very practical orientation that the healthcare professions have to their work. However, this chapter has argued that this is far from being the case, and that research and evidence-based practice are at the very heart of your practice. This chapter has also suggested that research is not only easy to understand but that you already understand it and practise it. Research drives practice to become ever better at delivering care to sick people. Research is not as clearly visible as 'orthopaedics' or 'surgery'; this is because research actually underpins everything that healthcare practitioners do. In this way, to find research, one needs not to look around oneself but rather to look at the ground upon which practice is standing.

Summary

- It is easy to be blind to the research happening around us, but examples of research affecting practice are everywhere; we only need to look.

- The healthcare professions are all 'practice' disciplines. Their rightful orientation is the care of the patient. Research has exactly the same orientation and is performed by practitioners exercising the same orientation they had as students – that is, to improve patient care.

- Research is an eminently practical and focused activity.

- The principles of research are easy to understand. You are already familiar with research, and you practise it in your daily life as an intelligent student with great potential. This chapter has tried to persuade you to look at research in a new light, but it has not had to 'teach' you anything.

- Your goal at this point in your career is to become a skilled practitioner, to be accepted by the healthcare team and to have developed a sense of mastery over the clinical field in which you will choose to work. Your goal is entirely appropriate and creditable. However, there will come a time when you will want to exercise your duty to your profession as a whole and to help people all over the world deliver better care. This is an orientation that you should begin to foster now. Being involved in research is one way in which you can make a difference on such a scale as this.

Further reading

Andresen, E. M., J. J. Tang, *et al.* (2006). 'The importance of occupational therapy contributions to health services research'. *OTJR: Occupation, Participation & Health* **26**(3): 108-116.

Fessele, K. (2007). 'Behind the scenes of clinical research: from trial to triumph'. *ONS Connect* **22**(8): 8-12.

Smith, M. C. (2007). 'Nursing research: what is it and how can dermatology nurses use it?' *Dermatology Nursing* **19**(5): 435-438.

Snow, T. (2008). 'Is nursing research catching up with other disciplines?' *Nursing Standard* **22**(19): 12-13.

Taylor, L. and J. Copeland (2006). 'Changes in physiotherapy research, education and professional development in New Zealand'. *Physical Therapy Reviews* **11**(2): 101-105.

Winsett, R. P. and A. K. Cashion (2007). 'The nursing research process'. *Nephrology Nursing Journal* **34**(6): 635-643.

References

Austin, L. (1988). 'The salt bath myth'. *Nursing Times* **84**(9): 79.

Baskett, P. and D. Zideman (2005). 'European Resuscitation Council Guidelines'. *Resuscitation* **67**(Supplement 1): 1-190.

Canning, D., J. P. Rosenberg and P. Yates (2007). 'Therapeutic relationships in specialist palliative care nursing practice'. *International Journal of Palliative Nursing* **13**(5): 222-229.

Charters, A. (2000). 'Wound glue: a comparative study of tissue adhesives'. *Accident & Emergency Nursing* **8**(4): 223-227.

Helberg, D., E. Mertens, R. J. G. Halfens and T. Dassen (2006). 'Treatment of pressure ulcers: results of a study comparing evidence and practice'. *Ostomy Wound Management* **52**(8): 60.

Kieslich, C., G. Marquardt, G. Galow, R. Lorenz and G. Jacob (2001). 'Neurological and mental outcome after severe head injury in childhood: a long term follow-up of 318 children'. *Disability and Rehabilitation* **23**(15): 665-669.

Meyers, T. A., D. J. Eichhorn, C. E. Guzzetta *et al.* (2004). 'Family presence during invasive procedures and resuscitation: the experience of family members, nurses, and physicians . . . reprinted with permission from the *American Journal of Nursing*, 2000; 100(2): 32-42'. *Topics in Emergency Medicine* **26**(1): 61-73.

Rognstad, M. and O. Aasland (2007). 'Change in career aspirations and job values from study time to working life'. *Journal of Nursing Management* **15**(4): 424-432.

Walsh, M. and P. Ford (1989). *Nursing Rituals, Research and Rational Actions*. London: Heinemann.

Wigert, H., R. Johansson, M. Berg and A. Hellström (2006). 'Mothers' experiences of having their newborn child in a neonatal intensive care unit'. *Scandinavian Journal of Caring Sciences* **20**(1): 35-41.

Windich-Biermeier, A., I. Sjoberg, J. C. Dale, D. Eshelman and C. E. Guzzetta (2007). 'Effects of distraction on pain, fear, and distress during venous port access and venipuncture in children and adolescents with cancer'. *Journal of Pediatric Oncology Nursing* **24**(1): 8-19.

Chapter 2
The literature: looking at what we already know

CHAPTER OBJECTIVES

The objectives for this chapter are to:

- Differentiate professional literature from other, less formal, literature

- Recognise the rationale for using the professional literature in preference to other forms of writing

- Be able to locate the professional literature

- Clarify the meaning of description, analysis and synthesis

- Begin to develop the confidence required to make sense of the professional literature, in part, by appreciating that the reader's skills in relation to their writing at this level are already well developed.

Chapter outline

Research is a very practical activity. However, you could be excused for thinking that research exists only as a great deal of written material, much of it both long and complex. This chapter aims to clarify the purpose of the professional and research literature and how it fits in with the ethos of professional practice.

This chapter will argue that, although the healthcare disciplines do have a clear practice orientation, the professional and research literature is necessary for them to develop and to progress. This chapter will look at the differences between the professional and the research literature, how to find the literature and how to make sense of it.

Just a thought

Are you a typical student? It does not take long for students (and staff) to realise that the Internet can be a very useful tool. Answers to almost any question can be found easily, using one of the freely available search engines. In fact, the search engine and the Internet itself have become such an integral part of the computer that it is hard to imagine the point of a computer without these facilities. So, it is not surprising that students today use their Internet search engine (e.g. Google®) where, years ago, students would have used the university library. Indeed, it is probably the case that some students have yet to find their way to the library, with its intimidating edifice, complicated catalogue and knowledgeable librarians. The university library can be an intimidating place.

It is common sense that directs students to what seems to be easily the best source of knowledge: the Internet search engine. However, from time to time, it may be better to turn your computer off for a while and go to your university library. Here's why.

There are some very special people found in a university library – other students. These students don't talk, they don't eat and they are never seen to drink beer. These students are studying; they are focusing their whole mind on one single activity. There is silence except for the sound of the occasional dusty volume being moved from shelf to table. There is an atmosphere here that is conducive to study. Here, in the library, there is a strange, if not decidedly odd, camaraderie of fellow students, though communication between student and student is limited to the occasional eye contact, grimace or smile. This is powerful stuff; not only do essays get written in double quick time but it has been known for life-long relationships to be formed in the library, grown up from all that eye contact and from the grimaces and smiles indicative of a common understanding. So, be wary of the library: you may get your essay written ten times faster than if you used Google at home, and you could also end up with a friend to carry your essay home for you.

Research is just common sense. In this, it is no different from dealing with any other everyday challenge. It follows that science that is grounded in research is just common sense too. Research is about questioning; it is about those situations where we are not sure we have an answer. However, not everyone questions; you may know people whose lives are chiefly orientated to 'doing the right thing', to complying with the rules set by others and for whom wondering and working things out for themselves seem never to be part of their lives. So let us be clear: although research is simply common sense, it is not for everyone. To be involved in research, even to take it seriously, one needs to be prepared to wonder, to ask questions and to have sufficient confidence in yourself to believe that you can make a difference.

It is perhaps too easy to think that there must be someone out there who knows the answer to a question or that there are others who will sort out a problem for us. Research is for those of us who are prepared to question, prepared to believe that our views and our intellectual skills are valuable and that we can and should use these skills to contribute to the common weal.[1]

It has already been made clear that you are not just anyone. In fact, you are a very special person. You are prepared to challenge yourself through your study and practice so that you can practise effectively and make a difference to people's lives. There are times in this process when you will simply absorb the knowledge that other people possess. However, your profession is not just a job; it is made up of people with a 'professional' orientation, which in part means that they accept an obligation to make a unique contribution to your discipline. In other words, you are a wondering, questioning, person. You already possess the confidence to know you can make a unique contribution to your discipline. You respect those people with more experience and knowledge than yourself, but at the same time you believe you can contribute to the knowledge base of your discipline, improve it, make it better; importantly, you intend to do just that in the years to come.

It is important to understand the points made here, because in this chapter we will begin the search that is 're-search'. In doing this we will not ask ourselves why we should bother or why we can't simply ask a more experienced person to tell us the answer to our question.

Searching the existing literature is near the beginning of the research process. Here, we want to find out what has already been written on the subject. We want to understand what is already understood by others and what research has

---

[1] *Common weal* means for the good of everyone.

already been completed on the subject in question. In searching the literature, however, we are not content to find out what that literature contains. Rather, we intend to use this knowledge to create more knowledge through research. We are motivated to do this for one very simple reason: we wish to contribute to that body of knowledge, to add to it through our own intelligence and endeavour. We are thus motivated because we are determined that, in our working life as a practitioner, we will make a difference.

Why look at the existing literature?

Research is a significant investment. Most research projects cost money and take a considerable amount of time to complete. It is necessary to make sure that we do not waste our time by, for example, conducting a study that may already have been done by someone else.

There is more than one way of conducting a study. Research techniques, or methodologies, are developing all the time. It makes sense to look at how other people have conducted their studies to find out which methodologies are most successful in different circumstances.

Research is designed to do just one thing - that is, to build on the discipline's body of knowledge. This building should be cumulative and organised. If we were building a house, it would be no use building the ground floor before we had built the foundations, and so it is with research. So, we need to know what research has already been done, so that we can build on it in a logical (common-sense) and ordered manner.

It is sometimes necessary to find out what is *not* known and what has *not* been researched so far. Sometimes, people have a new idea and they wish to initiate a completely new line of enquiry. Even here, the researcher will need to search the literature to be sure that his or her idea really is new. It is in the nature of things that this is a relatively unusual position in which to be. However, practice has made use of qualitative research to explore new understandings of the experiences of patients and clients (Terry and Carroll 2008). In fact, healthcare practice is quite good at using novel and flexible approaches in research. Healthcare practitioners seem also to be good at focusing their research on the lived experiences of patients and clients and even other staff (Chung *et al.* 2005). In these situations it is not uncommon for whole new lines of enquiry to be initiated. Even here, it is still important to be aware of what (if any) research has been completed on the subject in question and to be aware of the methodologies used to achieve both the collection and the analysis of data. All this requires a search of the existing literature to take place.

What is 'the literature'?

We need to recognise that there is a difference between the content of most web pages and what exists as the professional literature. Let us be clear about what it is that constitutes the professional literature.

Professional literature:

- is written using an accepted standard of language that is respectful of other professionals, even when criticising their work (Happell 2008);

- employs language that is non-emotional and is objective rather than subjective;

- is focused on the subject in question;

- contains both analysis and synthesis. The result is an objective and systematic exploration of the matter in question. Synthesis is to accept the challenge set by conflicting sets of information. It is never sufficient, for example, to write that one research project suggests one thing and another suggests something else – somehow, coherent sense needs to be made of the conflicting information;

- is made subject to peer review: no professional material is published without being judged by the author's peers. This peer review process is anonymous: the reviewers do not know the identity of the author and, in responding to the reviewers' comments, the author is not aware of the reviewer's identity. It is in this way that the written material is judged on its own merits and not on the past achievements or reputation of the author.

All professional literature complies with the criteria listed above. In confining our search to the professional literature, we rule out:

- many books, especially those that are aimed at telling us how to do things;

- most of the magazines you can find in a newsagent's shop;

- most web pages and most of the material that can be found by an Internet search engine.

However, finding the professional literature has never been easier, at least for university students with access to online databases.

At this point, we need to note that there are essentially two kinds of professional literature. The first is sometimes called 'anecdotal', which simply means that it is not research. This is not a lower class of literature; it is just that professionals and academics write about all manner of things and do not confine their work to research. This anecdotal literature complies fully with our criteria, but it isn't research. It follows that the second kind of professional literature is that based on research. Typically, when a research project is completed, the research team will publish the research, so that others can read it and be aware of the results of the study. It is important for us to be able to distinguish between anecdotal and research literature. Here, we are interested in research and the knowledge and evidence that research produces. We may use the anecdotal literature for ideas and for background reading, but most of our attention will be confined to the research literature.

It is easy to tell the difference between anecdotal and research literature. One is not research and one is research. However, students do sometimes confuse the two. A single journal may publish both kinds of material. Anecdotal literature can be, and often is, searching, critical and analytical, and it may consider existing research. Sometimes students confuse a published literature review with research because the authors have researched the topic. Real research, however, involves collecting new data or at least performing a new analysis on data.

Anecdotal literature is not less worthy than research literature. Anecdotal literature performs an essential role in professional life. However, it does represent a lower level of knowledge than does research. In practice, when we search the literature to inform a research project that we intend to undertake, we are interested mainly in the research literature – that is, what research has been done before, how it was done, how successful it was and what new information it produced.

Embedded in these criteria for professional and research literature are the foundations of science itself. These criteria are so important that they have created what we know as 'science'. However, there is no rocket science here. What distinguishes professional literature and scientific literature (which is much the same thing) from other forms of writing are criteria that can be readily understood and that are common sense.

So, if this is science, what is art? In what way is the study of English literature, for example, different from scientific writing? The distinction between science and the academic study of art does seem quite unclear. Perhaps it is not for nothing that English literature and science can both be studied at university; they are both intellectual disciplines. Perhaps the distinction between the academic study of art and that of science does not really add up to much. So, perhaps the use of the term 'professional literature' rather than 'scientific literature' is appropriate. It is certainly the case that academics who write professionally about Dickens's books, for example, will employ all of the criteria listed above. Perhaps science itself is something of a fabrication; certainly, there seems to be confusion about what exactly it is. However, what is important here is that we are clear about the meaning of the term 'research'. Both the arts and the sciences conduct research, and the criteria they use for what they write is the same. This point is salient to the healthcare professions. Nurses, for example, do often find that they are more interested in the softer side of science. It is not surprising that nurses are often interested in human experience of pain, grief, psychiatric illness, parenting, illness and a thousand other interesting topics. We can perhaps now see that the distinction between art and science is not very useful.

Even if we were clear about what constitutes science, we could still not say that nursing is a science. Like medicine, nursing is a practice discipline, and the word 'practitioner' seems to suit nursing better than the word 'scientist'. Nursing is a field of practice; it is not a science. However, science can be and often is found in nursing. Nursing becomes scientific whenever a professional nurse seeks to address a topic using the criteria of respect for other professionals, objectivity, focus, and the collection and analysis of new data, and when that nurse seeks to publish his or her work by subjecting it to peer review.

So, perhaps we can begin to see the value of the professional literature. The professional literature is not just writing or published stuff. Actually, it has a value commensurate with the adoption of the criteria identified above. The adoption of these criteria sets professional literature aside from, if not above, much of everything else that is written. Much that is written in books and on web pages is both good and useful, but the professional literature is different. Furthermore, the research literature represents what is science in each discipline; in medicine, nursing, English literature and the history of art.

How do I trust the literature?

In practice, there is a hierarchy of quality in the professional literature. Books are usually at the bottom of the hierarchy because they tend to limit their content to description. In practice, there is very little research to be found in books. The research that does exist in books is usually limited to brief description of what research is available. This can come as a surprise to the new student because those outside professional life often consider books to be clever things. Maybe they are clever, but sadly very little research is found in books and so books seldom meet our purpose. Books are useful when it comes to describing things, such as when you are learning how to practise surgery. However, for evidence of real research, we almost always have to look to journals and to a subset of journals that are regarded as academic.

It is not uncommon for the whole notion of research to be dismissed by under-graduate students. After all, you will be aware of conflicting research. One study tells us one thing, and another study tells us something that conflicts with the first study. It is not unnatural to see this as evidence that research is untrustworthy. Let us look at the argument that research is valueless because of the way that one study so often disagrees with another study. Well, it's true: studies do often find evidence that contradicts earlier studies.

Research is not an infallible endeavour. Researchers are human beings; they may be clever but they are not perfect. Researchers don't always get every-thing right. More usually, however, researchers do manage to do the best they can with the resources available to them. It is just that some things are very difficult to research. Researchers usually do their best in such circumstances, but sometimes the circumstances defeat them.

Research should be, and usually is, a cumulative endeavour. One research project builds upon another. It is not at all unnatural that, at one point in time, the available research appears to be contradictory. In the fullness of time, we are able to see that the research was progressing towards a known goal. When that goal is achieved, the progress can be seen in perspective and it can be seen that the research was pushing forward the front line of knowledge. With each push, however, there often comes a backlash of evidence as areas of knowledge defend the onslaught. Perhaps it is like a battle. There are winners and losers and there are reputations at stake. Researchers are human and they will, and indeed they should, try to defend their position against the advance of new knowledge. New research, producing new knowledge, should not have it easy. Such new knowledge should be challenged and challenged again until there is nothing left to challenge, until we can be certain that the new know-ledge is right, correct, certain and that it should therefore replace the old knowledge. The point is that there is friction and challenge here, which does release energy. We should expect this and welcome it. For such friction is part of the advancement of new knowledge. Nothing else would be right; new know-ledge should be challenged and then it should be challenged again. We must be sure that what we know is correct and that it should rightfully replace the knowledge that has gone before.

Example from practice

Family-centred care has been a defining concept in paediatric nursing for at least the past 30 years. It is a mode of nursing that emphasises the status of the child patient as a member of a family and the role the family should always have in the delivery of medical and nursing care. The approach to nursing also emphasises the child's psychological, developmental and social needs, and the way that these are intimately related to the functioning of the family within which the child plays a central part. Shields *et al.* (2007) undertook a systematic review* of family-centred care to determine what evidence existed to support its continuing practice. However, the authors of the systematic review found that there were no existing studies of a suitable quality. Family-centred care is practised by most, perhaps all, paediatric nurses, and so it seems strange that no good-quality research exists on the matter. However, family-centred care is a collective term for a wide range of approaches to care, some of which are conceptual rather than practical. Paediatric nurses work with a large number of children, from babies to young adults, and a wide range of illnesses. In this way, family-centred care is probably unresearchable. Rather, it is necessary to research each individual aspect of family-centred care. Fortunately, evidence of this kind does exist. For example, Kain *et al.* (2007) found that the application of the principles of family-centred care did help children who were waiting for surgery. Nevertheless, the work by Shields *et al.* (2007) does illustrate the way in which some research may simply be impossible and (by implication) a lot of research may be very difficult to do well.

*A systematic review is a collection of the best research on a particular topic where an attempt is made to pool the data from all the studies and to analyse the new, larger pool of data. In this context, the word 'meta-analysis' is sometimes used.

So, we are not going to be put off by conflicting research and disagreement. However, there is such a thing as poor-quality research. It is often difficult for the student to judge what is good or not-so-good research. After all, most students have little or no experience of actually doing any research. To expect students to judge the quality of research is like asking them to judge the performance of a neurosurgeon or a deep-sea diver. Until one has gained experience of doing a job, one is not in a very good position to judge it. What makes this matter worse is that the research literature can be very difficult to understand, and inexperienced students will often deal with this by confining their search to the less academic (popular) journals. The inevitable consequence of this is that they stumble across the less-good research literature. It can be better to confine the search to the more academic journals. While this can yield up research papers that can be difficult to understand, at least one can be assured that the quality of the research is better than poor. The message is clear: don't shy away from the more academic, less popular, journals. Rather, try to read them, and then read them again until they begin to make sense. This is not easy but it is better to grasp the nettle rather than settle for less.

Most online databases, such as Academic Search Elite (EBSCO Host: **http://search.ebscohost.com**), will enable you to tick a box next to your search term to indicate that you are only interested in peer-reviewed articles (always tick this box, as in Figure 2.1). However, it is also possible to choose only those journals with an impact factor. The impact factor measures the number of times that articles in a particular journal are cited – that is, referenced within other publications. In this way, the impact factor is a measure of how used are the articles published within a particular journal. So, the impact factor is a measure of the quality of the journal, not the individual papers published by that journal. If you wish to take this route, you can decide to confine yourself to journals that have an impact factor or you can look at those journals with the highest impact factor. It can be useful to know which journals have the highest impact factor but, other than that, the baseline of peer-reviewed journal is sufficient.[2]

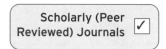

Figure 2.1 Ticking the box indicates that you're interested only in peer-reviewed journals.
Source: © EBSCO Publishing, Inc., 2009. All rights reserved.

Where do I find the professional literature?

Most people are used to using the Internet and are adept at using search engines such as Google® to find information. Google can be used to find information about almost anything, and it is a great resource. However, it isn't a good idea to use Google to search for literature, as there are better ways of doing this. Instead of using Google, try the variety of online databases that are purchased by your university and that are available on the Internet (online) and are usually accessed via university library web pages.

[2] If you want to know more about impact factors, find the *Journal of Citation Reports* on your university library web page.

If you are a university student, you will have easy access to these electronic journals and to online databases that do a great job of tracking down the material you are looking for. Things are much more difficult if you do not have this free access to the online journals. It is probably not enough to subscribe to just one journal. Today, there are so many journals that one journal cannot hope to publish all the best research articles. If you are not a university student, then it may be best to pay a subscription to just one of the online databases (there is a list at the end of this chapter). This will make available to you a whole raft of journals. Librarians have been particularly adept at keeping up to date with the changing style of library usage. Today, the average librarian possesses a wealth of knowledge about which online journals are available and which ones are best for which purposes. The average librarian has become an expert in the use of computers to access good-quality material via online databases and online journals. So the message is clear: use your librarian. This often involves meekly entering the ivory tower of the library, searching out a busy-looking librarian and admitting to being lost. Don't worry, we have all been there.

Now, the impatient librarian does exist. Today, the average librarian has degrees to spare. However, where a little respect is shown, the librarian will be keen to whisk the average student off his or her feet and wrap that poor student in arms of benevolent guidance. Being a student (and we never stop being one of those) is an exercise in resource management. Most students don't have much in the way of resources, and so the good use of what resources are available is much required. The librarian is the student's best birthday present – a free, knowledgeable and willing resource, a positive fountain of knowledge, there just to serve you. Use your librarian.

An example of a suitable online database is Cinahl (EBSCO Host: **http://search. ebscohost.com**). Using such a database is very easy. Simply enter your search string (e.g. 'pain AND child') into the search box and then (Figure 2.2):

- always tick the 'peer reviewed' box;

- select the 'publication type' to 'research'; options to search for particular types of research such as double-blind control trials may also be available;

- select the 'full text' option to save you much time in finding and ordering articles via your library;

- confine the date of publication to (for example) the past 5 years. This can be useful if you want the most up-to-date research and if leaving the option unticked results in too many articles being found.

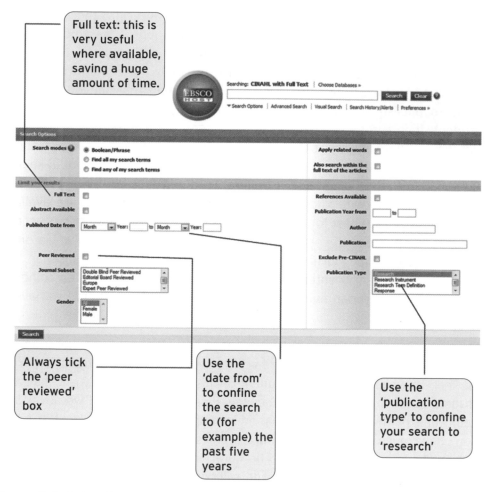

Figure 2.2 Using the Cinahl database.
Source: EBSCO Publishing, Inc., 2009. All rights reserved.

Figure 2.3 shows the first few results from our search for research on 'child AND pain'.

So, searching for and finding published research is easy. Increasingly, the databases to which university students have access contain the downloadable electronic version of published material. There is no good reason for failing to use these online databases.

Search engines such as Google do not tend to find the professional literature. They may find secondary references, but it will be more profitable to use one

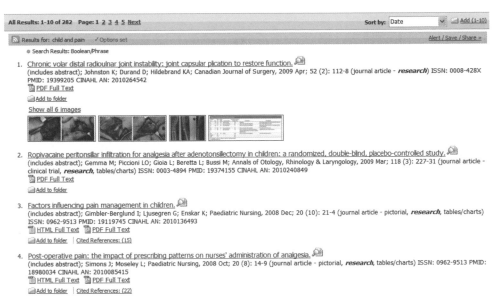

Figure 2.3 Search results for 'child' and 'pain'.
Source: EBSCO Publishing, Inc., 2009. All rights reserved.

of the web-based databases that are specifically designed to hold professional literature. As a student of a UK university (and most non-UK universities), you will not have to pay to use these databases. It takes no more than half an hour to become relatively proficient at using these databases. So, while the rest of the world is happily using Google, you should be surfing elsewhere.

In the past few years, another useful source of published research has become available: the Cochrane Library (**http://www3.interscience.wiley.com**) is essentially another online resource, but it focuses on systematic reviews and controlled trials (Greenhalgh 1997). Controlled trials can be found elsewhere (although the Cochrane Library is an excellent source), but the Cochrane Library is the best place to go for systematic reviews.

The Cochrane Library is becoming the single best source for research literature. However, it tends only to hold good-quality quantitative studies. It may be necessary to look elsewhere for more explorative or qualitative work.

For the student who is starting out on their journey into the research literature, the sources Cinahl and the Cochrane Library should prove sufficient. Between them you can find hundreds of thousands of research papers.

New words

Systematic review A relatively new form of research that collects together all the best research on a particular topic and attempts to make sense of the resulting collection of studies (Greenhalgh 1997). Often, a systematic review will pool the data from several studies and run an analysis, known as a 'meta-analysis', on the pooled data. Where successful, this effectively increases the sample size and can offer up new information that was not available by looking at each individual study. As such, a systematic review can constitute new research. Full access to the Cochrane Library will be available via your university library web page.

Randomised control trial (RCT) An experiment or prospective research study that has at least one control group and where randomisation is used to control bias. Blinding is also used in RCTs; this is where the participant and, perhaps, the researcher are not aware of the research group to which the participant has been allocated. Blinding helps to reduce the risk of bias. The RCT tries to mimic the archetypal laboratory experiment by controlling any variable that might impact on the research.

Making sense of published research

Research is easy to understand. Although it often looks complex, underneath all the apparent gobbledegook is something essentially very simple. So, when you look at your first research paper, you could be forgiven for thinking that this claim has been overstated. It is true that research does often look very complex. This is due in part to the language used by researchers and in part to the huge variety of research methods in use. Healthcare students are often more bewildered by research than are students of other disciplines such as medicine. The healthcare disciplines, like nursing and physiotherapy, are not pure disciplines, as are psychology or geography; rather, they are eclectic and diverse. Because of this, the healthcare disciplines employ a huge range of research methodologies, embracing as they do both the qualitative and the quantitative paradigms.

Part of the problem here is that a complicated research paper can make the average student feel inadequate, perhaps even stupid. It is still a good idea to read the paper through several times and to get help from your tutor or lecturer.

Be prepared to find research papers difficult to understand, especially at first. Try not to be put off by this. Take your research paper to a nice quiet place such as a library and try to understand it. It might not be easy. You will probably need a dictionary to look up all the new words – but do it all the same. Don't worry if it takes you all day or all week – it will *not* mean that you are stupid. There is a learning curve here: you have to climb the steep edifice of that curve before it begins to flatten out a little. If you expect the task to be difficult, then you will not feel quite so threatened when it proves to be difficult.

Words – reminder

Qualitative Essentially, explorative research that deals with words rather than numbers.

Quantitative Essentially, research that deals with numbers.

You may need to read the paper several times, but eventually you will make progress and it will become a little more clear. Now take it to your lecturer. Whatever excuse you gave yourself for not doing so is just that: an excuse to protect your self-confidence. Understand that this will take courage – but do it all the same. Go with a list (written down) of things that you do understand about the paper and a list of things you don't understand. Tell your lecturer what you think you understand about the paper and then the things you don't understand.

The point here is that it is easy to feel overwhelmed by the apparent complexity of the average research paper. This is a normal reaction. It does not prove that you are stupid; it proves only that you are human. Treat the paper like an invading army, something to be both attacked and defeated. Have courage, know that your mind is as keen as anyone else's, be prepared for a struggle and for set-backs, but be determined to conquer that research paper. By the end of this process the research paper will be lying exhausted at your feet. It will be defeated, its complicated language will have been translated into plain English, its methodology will be exposed as nothing more than a common-sense way of finding an answer to the question at hand, and the analysis, that array of frightening numbers and words, will be seen for what it is – the result of a clear and logical exploration of the data.

The chapters following this will guide you through the process of making sense of research papers. For now:

- Make sure that you are looking at a research paper. The paper should contain an analysis of data. The data may be numbers (quantitative) or words (qualitative), but there should be new information there, derived from a data collection. Don't confuse research with a literature review, even where this reviews previous research.

- Try not to use secondary papers (reports of other people's research).

- You will be used to critiquing things; however, try to go beyond criticising the researchers for what you think they have got wrong, because:

  - the people who published the research know more about it than you are likely to do; in criticising them, you may simply be exposing your own lack of understanding;

  - the main reason for research being imperfect is that some things are just very difficult to research. It is often impossible to use the most robust methodologies. For example, qualitative research is sometimes criticised for not coming close to the standards for a double-blind controlled trial, as used in most medical drug research. However, there are times when only the explorative nature of qualitative research will yield up the information that is being sought. Students new to research often fail to understand the real-world difficulties and constraints of research. People new to research often criticise researchers for failing to do what is, in fact, impossible. Such criticism is likely to do nothing more than expose the student's lack of understanding.

- Be sure that you report what the study found – that is, the results and not just the methodology (how the study was done). Make sure that you understand the results. If you are not sure how to interpret the results, read the paper again and then read it again, looking up all the words and phrases with which you are unfamiliar. If you still don't understand the results, ask your lecturer to interpret them for you.

- Make sure that you comment on the implications (as you see them) of the study. There will be implications for further study and for practice.

It is easy to be too descriptive when reviewing a research paper. You need to go beyond summarising it. Your report should have your ideas in it. There will need to be some description in your work, but there should also be an account of your ideas. Your section on the implications of the study is an excellent place in which to document some of your own ideas, your own thoughts and your own arguments.

Another thought – why do students write so many essays?

Let us understand this – students do not write essays so that they can be tested on the amount and depth of their knowledge. There are better ways of testing knowledge and it would be unforgivable to cause so many hours of work and the use of so many trees (paper) just to test students' knowledge and understanding. If we wanted only to test students' knowledge and understanding, we could simply talk to them, as in a viva, or give them a written examination with short-answer questions. Just think of the time and paper that would save. No, the rationale for the use of essays lies elsewhere.

An essay is an exercise in professional communication. An essay is the student's version of a published paper. It is about the same length as a published paper and it has the same characteristics as a published paper. These characteristics are that the essay:

- is written using an accepted standard of language;

- uses a discussion and arguments that are non-emotional and objective rather than subjective;

- is focused on the subject in question;

- 'tells a story': it contains a thesis – that is, a logical and integrated set of ideas that have a purpose, perhaps to inform the reader of something new or to enable the reader to see something in a new light. In achieving this, there is evidence of analysis and of the synthesis of existing and new ideas. In this way, the essay is a communication that goes way beyond summarising what already exists in other people's work. The essay is all about the student's own ideas;

- is made subject to assessment.

You have seen this list before, in the criteria for professional literature. So it is that in writing essays the student learns about writing professionally. Communication (sometimes in writing) is a requirement of professional life. Writing professionally is a vital component of both practice and research. There would be no point in improving practice or in conducting research if we then kept this new information hidden from others. We have a duty to publish our efforts, so that others can examine them, judge their worth and, where appropriate, incorporate the new knowledge into their own research and their own practice.

The use of analysis in the literature

Taken literally, the term 'analysis' means breaking something down into its component parts for the purpose of understanding them better. In practice, analysis is the sense that we make of things. It is often the case that, when we examine something, we have to pare away the irrelevant material so that we can see the relevant stuff more clearly.

Let's use the example of individualised care and the difficulties that exist in implementing it. Let's say that we want to examine the degree to which individualised care is something that is seen as positive and useful by patients and clients of the NHS. Let's look at some of the component arguments:

- Patients appreciate a healthcare service that adapts to their own needs

- Patients are irritated by a service that seems to be more about the needs of the institution than their own needs

- The public expects higher standards of care than in the past. As part of this, people expect their individual wishes and needs to be accommodated by the staff

- Healthcare practitioners provide care to individuals. Such a one-to-one orientation is certainly something that practitioners should be encouraging.

These arguments are pretty convincing. However, do these arguments present the whole story? Can you think of some reasons against the use of individualised care? List them here:

(1) ....

(2) ....

(3) ....

(4) ....

Here is what you may have written.

Individualised care is well and good, *but* it is just not realistic because:

- staff are too busy;

- staff don't have the time to modify every procedure for each individual;

- patients should be grateful for what is being offered – the NHS is a charity after all;[3]

---

[3] Actually, the NHS is not a charity, although it may manage charitable organisations and funds.

- if people want individualised care, they should obtain private treatment;

- staff don't work for individual patients: in practice, they work for a ward or unit. Staff work as a team. Their orientation to the ward, unit or department means that they work together with other people and so can't make individual exceptions to their care with every patient.

So here we have two sets of arguments in mutual opposition. We can't leave it like this, because we have to do something; we have to operate in one direction or another; we have to practise individualised care or generalised care.

We are not short of evidence; we have all the evidence here. What we are short of is analysis and synthesis. In analysis, we separate out the various arguments or components. In synthesis, we create a new position. By collating the various arguments and by categorising them (in this case, into 'for' and 'against' groups) we have achieved an analysis; in short, we have broken down the issue into its component parts for the purpose of understanding them.

Synthesis? What synthesis? No one has ever asked me to put synthesis into an essay. The word 'synthesis' is often subsumed by the word 'analysis'. In this way, when people use the word 'analysis', they often mean analysis and synthesis.

Doing this analysis has made things clearer. We have two groups of people – staff and patients – who have a quite separate orientation to the provision of healthcare. Indeed, patients and staff are not working together; even their aspirations for what the NHS can provide are in conflict. However, let's firm up our analysis to make it clearer, more succinct and more focused.

- Patients are interested only in themselves; they want care that is focused on their needs. Patients appreciate that other patients also have needs, but their own core role is to obtain the healthcare provision that they need to get well. That is why they are in hospital or are receiving care. When well, these same patients may fill their life with helping others. Now, though, it is time for them to receive care. It is a question of focus and priority. The purpose of being in hospital is to receive the care that they (themselves) need.

- Staff are loyal to their ward or unit and to the team of people with whom they work. They are conscious of patients' individual needs but are chiefly orientated to the generalised care that is provided (to all patients) on their ward or unit. This is good-quality care and is made better through it being a team activity. This provides a system in which all patients receive a fair percentage of the time the staff have to offer and in a situation where resources are often short. To be clear, staff work for their ward or department; they do not work for any one patient.

So, this is an analysis of the situation. It is an analysis with which you are free to disagree. An analysis is not necessarily the truth. You may have a different analysis, but in forming this you would have to assemble some more evidence, or identify where the analysis here has been illogically construed.

So, perhaps this is interesting; perhaps it even sheds new light on your understanding of individualised and generalised care. Perhaps you have been practising for 1, 2 or 3 years but only now feel that you understand this issue. Well, if so, you will understand the use and the power of analysis.

So, what about synthesis? Perhaps you have written an essay that presents all the available arguments but does not come to a conclusion, except perhaps to say 'Here are all the available arguments.' Consider a student who has reviewed the available research on a particular topic and found that some of the research evidence is conflicting. Our student summarises the available research but fails to come to a conclusion because the research itself is contradictory. The world is full of contradictory evidence, but when it comes to the practice of healthcare we have to synthesise all of this conflicting evidence so that it makes sense so that, as practitioners, we know what to do. Synthesis is takeing separate elements and creating a new whole from those elements. Theory, as in 'a theory of child development', is constructed largely from synthesis. Let's have a go at synthesis with our individualised care issue.

We cannot deny that nurses practising generalised care have done a good job over the years. Such a system is efficient and makes good use of resources. In addition, staff like it; they like working for an institution (the ward or unit) rather than for individual patients, and they like being part of a team. However, times change and the public's expectation of healthcare has changed. Not only do patients want individualised care; it is also good for them because they get from the system just what they need. When, for example, they are fit to be discharged home, they go home and do not have to wait until their take-home drugs come up to the ward with all the other drugs, tomorrow lunchtime or teatime or maybe not at all. There are those who would like to see staff achieve a more professional orientation to their work. From this source has come care planning, problem-orientated records and the many graduate and post-graduate courses that now exist for health professionals. We have to decide whether healthcare is still institutionalised, whether it exists to serve the hospital or NHS trust, or whether it exists to serve the patient.

Tick only one box in the table below. When you were younger and anticipating your career, did you see yourself primarily:

Working for a hospital or NHS trust	
Working for an ill person	

So, in synthesising this issue, we find that we have to make a decision. We have to decide whether our core priority is the sick person or the NHS. We understand now that we cannot be wholly orientated to both the NHS and the patient. With this synthesis we have a new ideology, one that is wholly orientated to the care of just one individual, where responsibility cannot be diffused among the whole team and where the practitioner must always be clear what healthcare provision he or she is dealing with. The old-fashioned nurse, working for the ward, where patients either toe the line or get in the way, is (in our synthesis of this issue) a dinosaur in a passing age.

Just as with our analysis, this synthesis is something with which you can disagree. However, in order to challenge it, you must bring more evidence or demonstrate that the synthesis here has been illogically construed.

So, we analyse something by separating out its component parts to better understand them. We use synthesis to generate new ideas, to make new sense of the issue or phenomenon in question. This is how it is with your essays and that is exactly how it is with the analysis we see being used in research. It makes little difference whether research uses words or numbers; the data (the words or the numbers) are subject to analysis, just as the ideas in your essays are. So, you already understand analysis. When you write an essay, you question the material contained in your essay. In exactly the same way, when we collect data in research, we subject the data to questioning – that is, we analyse the data. Sometimes, research does not only tell us something we did not know before; sometimes it also helps us to build a new kind of understanding. We use this new kind of understanding to synthesise new theory. Perhaps you have already achieved this in your essays. Perhaps you have begun to add to what is already known with new ideas of your own. Such is synthesis and so it is that you may already be skilled at it.

However, just like your essays, research does not always result in a new synthesis; often we have to be content with knowing better what we already knew reasonably well before. New ideas – those that have not been thought of before – are rare, and the process of producing new theory is a gradual one.

How to review the literature

Here is a step-by-step guide to reviewing the literature:

1. Identify a clear objective – what exactly do you want to find in the literature?

2. Identify the best source of literature – where will you look?

3. Identify what kind of literature you are looking for:

    a. research;

    b. anecdotal (non-research literature);

    c. an existing review of the literature;

    d. books.

4. Identify what resources you have available, especially how much time.

5. Identify the academic level of journal at which you are aiming.

6. Get help if you need it: librarian, library guides, etc.

7. Make notes on everything you read; consider keeping only electronic notes.

8. For the research literature, try to identify:

    a. What was the aim of the research?

    b. What was planned to be done (the research method)?

    c. How it was done (the intervention or techniques such as interviews or questionnaires).

    d. What was found.

9. For anecdotal literature:

    a. What was the focus of the paper?

    b. What was described?

    c. What was the author arguing?

    d. How was the argument supported?

    e. Is their argument credible?

10. Be prepared to read and re-read your literature.

11. Summarise the main points in the literature that you have read.

12. When you write your own account, you will be making your own arguments, based on the literature. So plan:

    a. your introduction to the topic;

    b. the arguments you will try to make;

    c. how you can use the literature you have found to support your arguments;

    d. what your conclusions will be.

13. Try to use discussion (in your introduction), analysis and synthesis.

14. Try to make your discussion flow logically.

15. Note that editing your essay can take longer than writing the first draft.

16. Ask yourself:

    a. Is my account clear, is it understandable?

    b. Is my English clear?

    c. What am I arguing?

    d. Are my arguments logically ordered?

    e. Have I provided an analysis?

    f. Where the literature is complex or where it suggests different things, have I synthesised these?

    g. Is my account interesting?

    h. Does my account add something to the literature I have read?

Let's go through this list in just a little more detail.

Identify a clear objective – what exactly do you want to find in the literature?

When you review the literature, you need to know exactly what you are looking for. It is not usually a good idea to review all the literature on 'asthma'. Whether you are conducting the literature review with a view to conducting research or to write an essay, you will need to have a tighter focus than this. If you haven't decided on a tighter focus at this point, it can be reasonable to 'eyeball' the literature to see what topics relating to 'asthma' have been covered. Doing this will also give you a reasonable idea about what aspects of asthma are most often dealt with and the depth of knowledge that already exists.

Identify the best source of literature – where will you look?

It is almost always best to locate the literature using one of the online databases provided by your university. Your librarian will help you choose the best one(s) for your subject area. Do make your search systematic. Makes notes on the search terms you have used. Looking at these notes will often lead to the use of other potentially useful search terms.

Identify the type of literature

You will find the following types of literature:

- research;
- anecdotal (non-research literature);
- an existing review of the literature;
- books.

It is unlikely that books are going to prove useful here but there can be exceptions to this. Other, more pure, disciplines such as sociology and psychology make much more use of books for their academic and research literature than do the healthcare disciplines. In healthcare, books tend to reflect 'knowledge', as in a summary of what is known on a particular subject. As such, books can sometimes provide useful background reading.

Our clearly defined focus for the literature review will tell us whether we need to be looking at the research or the anecdotal literature. In practice, the anecdotal literature should not be overlooked as it often contains non-research forms of evidence such as benchmarking and clinical experience. This level of evidence should be taken seriously, but we do need to be aware that research generally provides us with a superior level of knowledge about a given topic.

An existing review of the anecdotal or research literature can be very useful. Such a review never 'does the job for us' but, rather, it takes us on to a new level of enquiry. An existing review of the literature may well point to areas that still need to be explored and, as such, can provide the impetus to refine further what we want to achieve with our own review of the literature.

Example from the literature

Waldron, S. K. (2011). 'Auditory sensory impairments and the impact on oral healthcare: a review of the literature.' *Canadian Journal of Dental Hygiene* **45**(3): 180-184.

Waldron reviewed the literature of hearing impairment on oral healthcare. Waldron used the literature review to develop ideas on good practice and also to expose areas where future research could be useful; that is, where gaps in knowledge currently exist.

Identify what resources you have available

Whatever level and kind of literature review we are doing, we will be limited by the available resources. For UK university students, funding should not normally be an issue because students will have free (already paid for) access to online journals and full text databases. However, 'time' will tend to be a much more important issue. Available time is an issue for students who have one semester to write an essay, for PhD students who have 3 years to write their thesis and for researchers in receipt of a large grant. In the case of a typical university student, there will not be sufficient time within a semester to seek literature using the interlibrary loan facility. Most students should be content to use the full text facility of their university's online or library databases. This will allow access to an incomplete, yet still vast, amount of literature.

Identify the academic level of literature you wish to access

Anyone reviewing the literature should bear in mind the academic level of each of the journals in their discipline. There can be good articles published in the less academic journals but, as a general principle, the better-quality articles are found in the more academic journals. Your librarian will be able to help in identifying which are the more academic journals in your subject area. It is the case, however, that articles in the less academic journals do serve a useful function in professional life and tend to be written in a more 'accessible' language. If you are a new student, you may wish to limit your attention to these journals, at least for the time being.

Get help if you need it

When researchers are embarking on a new research project, they will often ensure that there is a librarian on their research team. Librarians are a great resource. Your tutor or lecturer should also be able to help. A typical university will have perhaps 20,000 students or more. It should not be necessary in such a situation for a student to have to struggle along on their own. Why not arrange to meet with other students, work together, share what you know?

Make notes on everything you read

It is easy to think that we will remember what we have read. We may also not want to have to do 'any more work' by writing notes on what we are reading. However, there isn't any way that any of us can remember everything we have read. If we don't make notes, we will find ourselves having to read the article again when we come to write the literature review. So, making notes on every-thing we read will save us time in the end.

It is no use making notes if the notes are likely to get lost or if they are so rambling that, at a later date, we are not able to make sense of them. We all suffer from 'disorganisation' sometimes, but being organised with notes is important because, if we are organised, we will save time and get the job of doing that literature review completed more efficiently.

Some people prefer to write their notes manually. However, it can be difficult to 'file' paper notes in such a way that they can be found again easily. Let us be clear – there is no point in making notes if the notes are then going to get lost. To deal with this issue, some people use one big 'diary' in which they keep all their notes. Other people keep a card index file. For me, neither of these options would be suitable. For one thing, my writing is awful – I can hardly read it. Your writing may be better than mine, but when you are tired, you too still may end up with some very untidy notes. A card index file is good if you like to spend your time cataloguing, but it is bulky and you won't have it with you when you need it. You may wish to keep your notes as word processor files and, in my experience, this works much better.

For me, however, the very best way of managing notes is to use 'reference managing' software. This is software designed specifically for managing refer-ences and for recording notes about articles. Such applications include EndNote and ProCite, and it is very likely that your university provides access to one or more of these applications. I used one of these applications to organise my notes and my references for this book. You can see some of these in the image below.

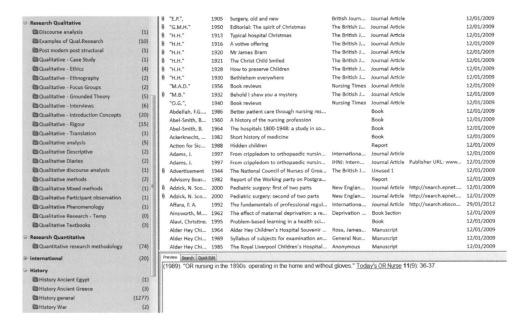

Here, you can see my references for the qualitative research chapters for this book. You can see that these references are organised according to their main focus. However, I can also search for any text in any of the references and I can assign a reference to several categories or classifications.

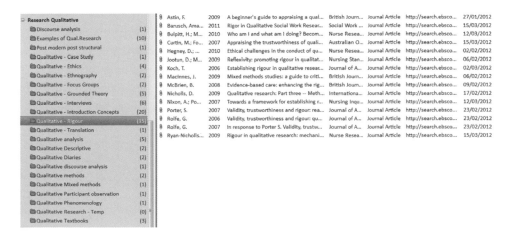

In the image above, you can see my reference for 'rigour' in qualitative research. Clicking on one of the references will open a page on which I can detail the actual reference and make notes on it.

Author
Bulpitt, H.
Martin, P. J.

Year
2010

Title
Who am I and what am I doing? Becoming a qualitative research interviewer

Journal
Nurse Researcher

Volume
17

Issue
3

Pages
7-16

Start Page

Here are my notes on the article by Bulpitt and Martin that I have used later in this book. Applications such as this one also allow for the references to be downloaded from the online databases and put directly (cited) into a word processor file. This produces an automated reference list which is always formatted correctly. Some of this software is web-based, so that it is possible to access one's file of references from anywhere where there is internet access.

Research Notes

Describes reflexive methodologies as a way of making qualitative processes transparent. Basically, the author is reflecting on his experience of interviewing for the first time (that's it, that's reflexive methology).

Does discuss his experience of interviewing for the first time.

9
Relates the interview as a similar experience to counselling.

Interviewing needs:
The ability to focus on the issues
Ability to listen
Good memory
Curiosity
Ability to establish a good raport.
Empathy.

Interviewers can influence the data that is collected.
Reflexive approach helps the researcher to identify bias in him or herself - develop 'an understanding of self in context'.

11
The difficulty of differentiating the research interview from a therapeutic interview. Argues that the aims of both are entirely different, one aims to heal and the other to understand (not sure I agree that the two are always so easy to separate; empathy requires at least a wish to heal).

14
Seductiveness - the interview may lead the participant to disclose something they ultimately regret disclosing.

URL
http://search.ebscohost.com/login.aspx?direct=true&db=rzh&AN=2010638177&site=ehost-live
Publisher URL: www.cinahl.com/cgi-bin/refsvc?jid=807&accno=2010638177
File Attachments

50369041.pdf

You can see that I have identified the page number to which each note refers and that some of my notes simply summarise a key part of the text, while other notes are a record of my own views of the text. You may also have noticed that I am able to keep a link to the pdf of the whole article.

It is much easier to write your literature review using notes. If you try to write the essay using a large pile of the original articles on your desk, the following will happen.

- You will tend to end up with an overly-descriptive account of the articles.

- Your account will tend to be too 'close' to the content of the articles; there will not be a lot of 'you' (your own ideas) in your literature review. This is because 'notes' are in part used to develop your own ideas.

- It will take you much longer to write your literature review than if you were able to work from your notes.

What notes to make

For the research literature, try to identify:

- What was the aim of the research?

- What was planned to be done (the research method)?

- How was it done (the intervention or techniques such as interviews or questionnaires)?

- What was found?

For anecdotal literature:

- What was the focus of the paper?

- What was described?

- What was the author arguing?

- How was the argument supported?

- Is the argument credible considering the literature the author used to support the arguments made?

You should also note:

- anything interesting;

- any views you have and any ideas you may have about the development of a new argument.

Remember that you are reading the literature because you want to find out what has already been done, what knowledge already exists. However, you are also reading the literature because you want to develop plans for your own work. For this reason, you should record any developing ideas for your own work that may be 'sparked-off' by the literature you are reading.

Be prepared to read and re-read your literature

If you have ever re-read a novel, you will probably have been surprised at just how much of the novel you missed the first time you read it. When you first read an article, you will probably be seeking to understand it, to develop a 'summary' of it inside your head. When you read it again, you do not have to do this, and so you are able to focus your mind on deeper aspects of the article.

Writing your literature review

Your literature review should be more than just a summary of the existing literature. Like a good novel, your own work should have a trajectory of its own. Your literature review should take the reader somewhere; you should be reviewing the literature for a reason, with a purpose in mind. In a research study, this purpose is usually to:

- be clear about what has been done before;
- lead the discussion toward where the literature takes us, what still needs to be researched.

So it is that the literature review in most research projects will lead directly to the methods section, the section that clarifies what the research intends to do and how it intends to do it.

When you write your own account, you will be making your own arguments, based on the literature. So plan:

- your introduction to the topic;
- what arguments you will make;
- how you can use the literature you have found to support your arguments;
- what your conclusions will be. These will be expressed in terms of your developing ideas about the research question and chiefly:
  - what still needs to be researched;
  - what, specifically, will be the proposed research question;
  - what will be the most suitable methods to achieve the desired result.

Try to use description, analysis and synthesis.

- **Description** – to clarify what research has already been undertaken and to summarise the literature

- **Analysis** – to interpret or judge the 'worth' of the material and how relevant it is to your developing research question or the key trajectory of the argument you wish to make

- **Synthesis** – to deal with unanswered questions. In research, it is often the case that two or more research projects seem to have conflicting 'findings'; it is necessary to 'deal' with this and to make judgements on what may cause this conflict. In the same way, different ideas on an issue discussed in the literature should be 'dealt with'. This involves weighing those ideas (arguments) in the 'balance' and coming to an overall conclusion (a synthesis) about them.

Try to make your discussion flow logically. The literature review is an exercise in communication. You are trying to communicate something that is very complex, in a manner that is coherent and logical. The literature review may be clever and technical but it should nevertheless read like a good novel. It should have 'a beginning, a middle and an end' and it should tell a story – a story of the development of your key idea or your research question.

Researching, designing and writing the literature review is a lengthy process. When it is written you will still have work to do. In fact, writing the literature review is the easy part of the process. Once written, the literature review must be read and read again. Read it to:

- identify faults in it;

- check that the discussion flows logically;

- check that your key argument(s) develop logically through the review and that they are pinned to the existing literature and are very clearly expressed at the end of the discussion;

- ensure that the literature review can lead logically to the development of the research question.

Conducting a literature review is very like writing an academic essay. The key difference is that the literature review has a clear purpose – it has a job to do. That job is: (1) to identify what knowledge on a particular topic already exists, what has been researched before and how it has been researched (what methods were used); and (2) to develop a new key idea, an idea that is capable of growing into a research question; a research question that will itself be the motivating force for a brand-new research study.

Concluding remarks

The research and professional literature exists as an essential part of practice and research. Not everyone likes to spend all their time reading. So, it is important to be able to search for the best literature quickly and to discern the salient points from that literature in a focused and efficient manner. In practice, the literature is the way in which both practitioners and researchers communicate their work to others. From the literature, we can see what is already known. Being informed of what is already known, we can begin the process of moving that knowledge base forward. No professional can be satisfied with the way things are; all professionals have ideas about how to make things better. The literature is the starting block for those ideas to be tested by research and for them to lead to new insights and new practices in patient care.

Summary

- The professional literature is different from less formal literature. Professional literature is written and published to a standard, where principally it is objective and made subject to peer review.

- The professional literature is not best accessed via Internet search engines, but rather exists in web-based databases such as that provided by Cinahl. It can also be found in university libraries where much expertise exists to help both the new student and the seasoned researcher to find information.

- The professional literature helps to define a profession. It is important because it is the main way in which professionals communicate their work and their research.

- The professional literature can be hard to understand. However, you are not only well on the way to being able to understand it and use it effectively; you are also advantaged in that you are pretty good at creating professional literature. The essays you have been asked to write during your course of study are the beginning of your publishing career. If you can write an essay, then you can write a paper and seek to get that paper submitted for publication.

- It is not enough to learn about your chosen discipline. No profession can survive on what people already know. It is necessary to make things better. You will want to have an active role in seeking out new knowledge. Having done that, you will want to tell everyone what you have found. Others will read what you have written because they will want to build on what you have achieved. They will look at the professional literature to find your work, and the result will be a profession that is always looking forward and always trying to improve what it can do for the people it tries to help.

- The literature review is an essential part of any research study. It serves the purpose of identifying (1) what has already been done and (2) what still needs to be done, what still needs to be researched.

Further reading

Cleary and Hunt clarify the process of searching for literature:

Cleary, M., G. E. Hunt *et al.* (2009). 'Conducting efficient literature searches: strategies for mental health nurses'. *Journal of Psychosocial Nursing & Mental Health Services* **47**(11): 34-41.

Cronin and Ryan clarify the process of reviewing the literature:

Cronin, P., F. Ryan *et al.* (2008). 'Undertaking a literature review: a step-by-step approach'. *British Journal of Nursing (BJN)* **17**(1): 38-43.

Note that it is usually best to access the following websites via your university library web page. If you try to access these sites from your home computer, you may find that you are denied access or are asked for payment. In practice, you will probably find that you have free access from your university computers and that your university computer centre staff will be able to tell you how to get the same free access from your home computer.

Ebscohost (for Cinahl and Academic Search Elite):

http://search.ebscohost.com/Community.aspx

The National Library for Health offers free access to the Cochrane Database (for systematic reviews and experimental research). The site also offers access to other databases that are normally paid-for resources:

http://www.library.nhs.uk/

References

Chung, B. P. M., T. K. S. Wong, E. S. B. Suen and J. W. Y. Chung (2005). 'SARS: caring for patients in Hong Kong'. *Journal of Clinical Nursing* **14**(4): 510–517.

Greenhalgh, T. (1997). 'How to read a paper: papers that summarise other papers (systematic reviews and meta-analyses)'. *British Medical Journal* **315**(7109): 672–675.

Happell, B. (2008). 'The responsibility of review: guidelines to promote professional courtesy and commitment through the peer review process'. *International Journal of Psychiatric Nursing Research* **13**(3): 1–9.

Kain, Z. N., A. A. Caldwell-Andrews, L. C. Mayes *et al.* (2007). 'Family-centered preparation for surgery improves perioperative outcomes in children: a randomized controlled trial'. *Anesthesiology* **106**(1): 65–74.

Shields, L., J. Pratt, L. Davis and J. Hunter (2007). 'Family centred care for children in hospital'. *Cochrane Database of Systematic Reviews* (1): CD004811.

Terry, L. M. and J. Carroll (2008). 'Dealing with death: first encounters for first-year nursing students'. *British Journal of Nursing* **17**(12): 760–765.

Waldron, S. K. (2011). 'Auditory sensory impairments and the impact on oral healthcare: a review of the literature.' *Canadian Journal of Dental Hygiene* **45**(3): 180–184.

Chapter 3
Evidence-based practice

CHAPTER OBJECTIVES

The objectives for this chapter are to:

- Provide a clear definition of evidence-based practice

- Show the relationship between evidence-based practice and research

- Identify the various forms of evidence that can be used to help develop practice

- Provide an overview of the basis of ethical research.

Chapter outline

Having identified the meaning of research in the previous chapter, we look now at the related concept of evidence-based practice. We will see that, although research may provide the best form of evidence (the best form of knowledge), there are other forms of evidence that are often used to support practice. This chapter will also look at some of the ways in which people sometimes avoid using evidence. The acquisition of evidence, through research or other means, must be carried out within the established principles of ethical conduct. This chapter will look at what this means for the researcher and for you, as you begin to make sense of a career within an ethical and evidence-based profession.

What is evidence-based practice?

Put simply, the term 'evidence-based practice' needs no interpretation: it is what it says it is – that is, practice based on evidence. However, there are two ways in which the term 'evidence-based practice' can be understood.

Meaning 1: the use of research as just one of many forms of evidence

It is possible to argue that there exists more than one form of evidence, with research being only one form or source of evidence. Research is arguably the best form of evidence, but there are reasons for the lack of availability of research in healthcare.

- Research is expensive. In Britain, there are no well-defined funding streams for research for nursing and healthcare disciplines other than medicine. Good-quality research usually involves the employment of research assistants, and this is usually very expensive.

- It is not always possible to conduct research to a recognisable standard. The healthcare professions work with people, and in some situations research with people would place them at risk or would infringe their human rights. Research with babies, for example, is problematic because it is not possible to gain the informed consent of the babies themselves and because responsible adults are limited in the degree to which they can consent for children where the research may not be in their child's interest. So, research is sometimes difficult or impossible to do, and good research that meets the accepted standard for control and randomisation is very often impossible to conduct within the arena in which health care practitioners operate.

In some ways, the use of alternative forms of evidence is justified. Where research conducted to scientific standards of control and randomisation is impossible, we have little alternative but to accept the use of research that does not meet these standards. In the same way, if research in any form is impossible, then there is little alternative but to accept other forms of evidence. Clearly, however, we need to insist on research evidence when such research is both possible and desirable, and we need to appreciate fully the dangers inherent in accepting forms of evidence that may be prone to error and that may be misleading.

The use of the term 'evidence-based practice' relates to an acceptance that forms of evidence other than that generated by research can be used appropriately. There is no universal agreement on such use of non-research evidence. However, healthcare is replete with examples of practice based on non-research evidence, and so it is important to give this area some thought, if only with a couple of caveats.

- Where research conducted to scientific standards remains achievable, other forms of evidence should always be seen as less than adequate.

- Non-research evidence should be understood to be particularly vulnerable to flaw and error and to possess a capacity to mislead.

In short, research evidence is almost always the best form of evidence, and healthcare practitioners should always seek evidence from research. However, other forms of evidence cannot be easily dismissed, may at the very least be interesting, and may all too often represent the best evidence available to us at the moment.

Meaning 2: a process by which poor or ineffective practices are weeded out and better practice is identified and implemented

The term 'evidence-based practice' is also used to denote practice that is based on some form of evidence, as opposed to practice that fails to be supported by any form of evidence. The term 'evidence-based practice' was probably first used in medicine and reflected an attempt to weed out practices that had a basis only in tradition and experience or to ensure that such practices were properly evaluated and made subject to peer review.

It was perhaps the early use of the term 'evidence-based medicine' that encouraged the use of non-research forms of evidence. This was not because these forms of evidence were in any way considered superior to research but that *any* form of evidence was an evolutionary move in the right direction. Just to get medical practitioners to think about their practices and to look at what other practitioners were doing was a major and very important step forward for medicine. In other words, we need to see evidence-based practice in evolutionary terms. Medicine and other healthcare disciplines are evolving, trying to improve. All healthcare disciplines have had to learn to stand before they could learn to walk, to look at their practice objectively before being able to subject it to research.

Non-research forms of evidence

Let's look at what other forms of evidence are sometimes used to support practice.

Peer review

Peer review is a central component of professional life and an important mechanism for ensuring that practice is supported by at least some form of evidence. Peer review can be applied to a new idea, a practice innovation, continuing professional registration, publication and just about every aspect of professional life.

A peer is someone like you - your equal. In this way, peer review for students would be undertaken by other students and not by academic or practice staff. Peer review for publication would be undertaken by people who are themselves nurses who publish their own work from time to time. Peer review in clinical practice is undertaken by other practitioners and not by managers or (usually) people from other professions.

Clinical audit

Clinical audit is, arguably, a form of research. However, it tends to be concerned with the collection of descriptive (as opposed to experimental) data, which have to do with documented standards of patient care. Audits do not usually achieve the standard of scientific research because they lack the necessary control of variables, and randomisation is seldom possible. Despite these failings, audits are used widely and do provide valuable feedback on measures of the quality of patient care.

Benchmarking

Benchmarking is a form of standard that is set by a community of practitioners, often by a local group of hospitals. A standard, or benchmark, is set, and work takes place to establish that standard and perhaps to exceed it. The power of benchmarking lies within the liaison that takes place within the community of practitioners. In the case of a local group of hospital staff, this community of practitioners might not have come together except for the purpose of establishing the benchmarking. So, benchmarking encourages liaison outside one's own workplace; it has the effect of first equalising the standard of care being practised in individual departments across a region or area and then improving that standard further. Benchmarking is a mix of both peer review and the development of standards. It has the advantage that the benchmark is set by practitioners rather than managers. In this way, the development or initiative is fully owned by the practitioners themselves.

Established clinical expertise

Healthcare practice is full of expert knowledge. Much of this knowledge has been acquired through experience. However, experience is best used when it is shared with others, debated in public and published. This offers the opportunity for other experts to point out possible flaws in relation to the practice in question.

Although clinical expertise falls short of what research is able to offer, it should be recognised that people know a lot of things that have never been subject to research. Clinical expertise is a valuable resource. However, knowledge can

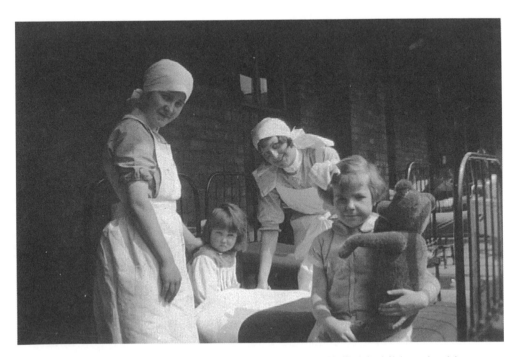

Figure 3.1 For most of the twentieth century, hospitalised children had to cope without their parents.

sometimes be more subjective than objective, and it is possible for lots of very capable people to believe that something is true when in fact it is not. There is a tendency for us to think that something must be right if everyone believes it, but it is possible for everyone to be wrong. For this reason, it is important that clinical expertise is made subject to close scrutiny and that it is evaluated objectively.

During much of the twentieth century, nurses did not allow parents to stay in hospital with their sick children (Figure 3.1). Sometimes, parents were not even allowed to visit their children, even when children were hospitalised for many weeks and when they were seriously ill (Jolley 2007, 2008; Jolley and Shields 2009). It was thought by almost everyone, nurses, doctors and hospital admin-istrators, that having parents in hospital with their children would cause the sick child harm (see Duncombe 1979). Only after the Second World War did people gradually come to appreciate that children had an important emotional bond with their parents and that having parents stay with children in hospital helped children considerably. So, just about everybody was wrong.

Tradition

'We always do it this way.' Perhaps you have been frustrated by a senior prac-titioner's desire to stick to the way things have always been done. Practitioners should be open to new ideas but so too do they need to recognise the wisdom of the past. If a particular type of wound has been dressed in a particular way for the past 50 years, then maybe there is good reason for continuing this practice. We may not have good evidence to support the practice in question, but neither may we have good evidence to abandon the practice. We have already noted that lots of people can be uniformly incorrect. Nevertheless, the more people who support a particular approach to care, the more likely it is that they are right. It is the case that they could all be wrong and it is definitely the case that global assumptions about good practice should be questioned and objective data sought. Nevertheless, tradition should not be dismissed too readily. Practices do not become tradition overnight and, although the process that selects them may be less than scientific and less than rigorous, processes designed to identify flaws almost always exist in these cases. It follows that traditional techniques have stood the test of time and do therefore deserve to be taken seriously. This notwithstanding, every practitioner (including you and me) has the right to challenge tradition. Tradition is fairly low down the hierarchy of knowledge and, as such, it should expect to be challenged, even by the most junior of staff.

Example from the literature and research

Western medicine is based on the principles of science and evidence-based practice. However, there are many parts of the world where western medicine has yet to develop or where it is in competition with traditional healing. The lack of evidence-based practice and research in traditional healing is often a cause for concern. However, the lack of evidence to support a particular practice does in no way mean that the practice is of poor quality. A lack of evidence simply means that we don't know whether something works. It follows that traditional practices should not be too readily dismissed. Xu *et al.* (2006) studied the practice of traditional healers in China who provide therapy for people with cancer. Their qualitative study found that patients did receive some benefit from the traditional healers. Indeed, the researchers suggest that this particular model of cancer care should be evaluated more fully to determine whether it could be of benefit as an adjunct to western medicine.

Experience

Experience is a little like tradition, except that it applies to only one individual. We should be careful before belittling experience, and yet it is a long way from the evidence produced by research. We have probably all come across situations where patients are treated differently, even on the same ward, because two consultants have been trained using two different techniques. It takes little thought to appreciate the need here to evaluate the two procedures, for one is likely to be superior to the other.

Experience is more credible if it is supported by others and especially if it is formally critiqued by peer review, as when someone attempts to publish an article promoting a particular practice. Publishing is important because the process of getting a paper published opens it to peer review (all the articles in the professional press are peer-reviewed before being published). Once the paper is published, it can be read and critiqued by a large number of practitioners. Publishing ideas on an example of practice both tells other people about those ideas and exposes the ideas to critique. In this way, publishing is an important mechanism of ensuring that practice is evidence-based and is an essential element of professional life. We should all publish because we should all have ideas about how practice can be improved.

> ## Example from the literature and research
>
> Stewart (2006) describes the development of new guidelines for catheterisation at a particular hospital. This paper describes the challenges that were overcome when peer review was used to ensure that the new guidelines were properly evidence-based and accepted by both the medical and nursing staff. The author illustrates how practitioners can themselves take ownership of a new initiative and can work together successfully to achieve a change in practice and to ensure that practice continues to be based on the best available evidence.

Policy and guidelines

Government develops health policy, and hospitals develop clinical standards of one sort or another. Mechanisms are often put in place to maintain practice within the parameters of the policy in question. In most cases, the policies are reviewed and audited to ensure that they continue to be appropriate and effective. Policies and the effectiveness of them can be compared between health institutions, even to the point where league tables can be formulated so that people can see which health organisations are performing best. These league tables are based on data, but these data often fall short of scientific standards. Even so, these data can be considered to be a form of evidence. An example of this form of evidence is the government's criteria for waiting times in accident and emergency departments. In this case, the government established a policy that hospitals should work to reduce waiting times. Accident departments were then audited to provide data on waiting times and the improvement or otherwise of waiting times. Using these data, it is possible to compare one accident department with other accident departments.

Policy formation can sometimes be politically charged. Clearly, the policies themselves relate to the prevailing political will (to reduce accident department waiting times). This is usually sufficiently transparent. However, the collection of data can also be politically motivated, largely because it is related so closely to the interests of agencies such as government and National Health Service (NHS) trusts (see Castledine 2008). It follows that care needs to be taken to ensure that bias has not influenced the data or their analysis. It might be possible, for example, to record patients as having been discharged from the accident department even though it is known that they have not yet been admitted to a ward or been taken home. Formal research can also suffer from bias. However, mechanisms are set in place to ensure that bias is properly controlled. Clinical audit and the evaluation of policy decisions often fail to implement these controls. In any case, it is always necessary to be wary of any data, the collection of which may be politically motivated or may serve the interests of a person or agency.

Research that does not meet the standard of scientific criteria

Many studies are published that use methodologies that are inexpensive to implement but that fail to provide the best forms of control and randomisation. Such studies may suffer from the effect of bias or from the effect of one or more variables that have not been properly accounted for. It is debatable whether these studies add much to our knowledge and evidence base. However, it is probably appropriate to consider them here as providing a form of evidence outside the parameter of fully fledged research projects.

Dyer (1997) considers the relatively high proportion of small-scale and poorly controlled studies in the nursing literature. However, rather than criticising these less-than-perfect studies, Dyer takes the view that they are part of the evolution of research in nursing and that they should be considered a legitimate source of evidence upon which practice can be supported.

Practice that is supported by anecdotal evidence and by the literature

Anecdotal evidence means non-research evidence. We have seen that the professional literature can usefully be divided into two categories: research and anecdotal. In common usage, anecdotal means unreliable or subjective; however, it really has neither of these qualities – it is just *not* research. A typical example of anecdotal literature is a nursing care study in which the author discusses the care given to a particular patient. The purpose of the study might be to tell the reader about a nursing initiative or to inform less experienced nurses about the care in this case and the implications that care had for one patient.

It should be clear that there is nothing at all wrong with anecdotal literature; in fact, much of the professional literature is anecdotal and it serves a very good purpose. Indeed, the anecdotal literature can be seen as the backbone of professional life. It is here that practitioners write about their initiatives so that others can learn from them and so for the express purpose of these initiatives being made open to critique by others. This is not research, but the combined effort of the original paper and the opportunity the rest of the profession has to critique that paper is as much evidence as anything else discussed here.

> ### Example from the literature and research
>
> Fiona Murphy (2006) published a care study in which she illustrated the use of a form of nursing assessment (Gordon's (1994) functional health patterns) to help focus nursing intervention on the needs of a young man requiring dialysis. The anecdotal discussion presents the case that Gordon's model has been useful. Murphy uses the discussion to propose the idea that nurses have an important and unique role to play in the care of people requiring dialysis. The paper does present evidence of both the usefulness of Gordon's model and of nursing's uniquely valuable role. By publishing this evidence in the professional press, Murphy is able both to present her case and to ensure that her arguments are made available for critique. It is these last two qualities that ensure the anecdotal discussion does constitute evidence.

The failure to use evidence

Intuition

Intuition is similar to the concept of an educated guess. A simple example of this is where a nurse accepts a new patient on to the ward. The nurse may want to collect a wide range of information from the new patient but this may take time. As a priority, the nurse ensures that he or she finds out just one piece of information – the patient's medical diagnosis. Our nurse takes the view that, with this information, he or she can plan care that is at least broadly appropriate. In this situation, the nurse is using intuition. The nurse takes the medical diagnosis and from this makes inferences about which nursing care is likely to be needed.

> ### Example from the literature and research
>
> Herbert *et al.* (2001) considered the view that evidence-based practice was simply too difficult to apply to the busy clinical arena. They considered the view that clinicians already knew what to do by virtue of their training, established practice, etc. However, after considering the arguments for and against evidence-based practice, they concluded that evidence-based practice did indeed have much to offer the clinical arena.

Too much reliance on intuition can work against the principles of evidence-based practice. Clearly, nursing is not medicine, and our nurse requires information on the patient's nursing needs to provide good-quality care. Intuition may be needed from time to time, perhaps in an emergency when there simply is not time to acquire all the information that we would like to have at our disposal. However, the overuse of intuition is an important cause of poor-quality care and it can drive nursing (and medicine) in the opposite direction from healthcare that is properly based on evidence.

Trial and error

Trial and error is perhaps the worst possible way to improve practice. By definition, this approach lacks methodology or any form of systematic planning. Trial and error involves dealing with a problem by randomly selecting a possible solution. If this solution seems to work, then it is adopted, without seeing whether another solution might work better. If no success is achieved, then the next possible remedy is selected and the process begins again. No attempt is made to see how other practitioners have dealt with the problem.

Trial and error is perhaps the easiest approach to use because it requires no effort. However, it is dysfunctional, resulting in wasted time and poor patient outcomes. It can never be fully successful. Even if one thinks that a good solution has been found, the possibility will exist that there is an even better solution out there somewhere. It follows that the best possible outcome of trial and error is a good-enough solution. Healthcare practitioners provide an important professional activity, and a good-enough solution can never be justified: it can never be good enough.

Unpublished endeavour

Let's consider a situation where an individual practitioner uses research to discover something new or a benchmarking group manages to improve an aspect of practice across several departments. Here, however, the individual researcher or the benchmarking group fails to publish their work. It follows that what has been achieved will not be made subject to review by a wider audience of practitioners, and practitioners everywhere will not be able to benefit from what has been achieved.

In a sense, the local initiative has managed to base its practice on evidence. However, this is not enough. Healthcare practitioners are professionals, which means that their responsibility does not start and end with the patient: these practitioners are responsible for the health and welfare of their profession and have a duty to ensure that knowledge is passed on.

Why is there not more published research in nursing and healthcare?

It is the case that nursing is a particularly broad (some might say poorly focused) discipline with a history outside mainstream academia. It is involved with modalities of traditional care, treatment for those with ill-health and trauma across all age groups and in both institutional and community-based health programmes, the prevention of ill-health and the promotion of health, including psychological, physical and developmental health. In addition, nursing probably still has an image of being an adjunct to medicine rather than an independent professional activity. Funding bodies naturally like to be clear about where they are spending their money. Medicine, with its tight focus on treating disease, presents an easily understood image to the organisations with money to spend on research. Perhaps it is the case that nursing needs to be clearer about what it does and what it aims to do, and much clearer about how it presents its image to the general public.

It is worth thinking about this a little more. Imagine the last time you came back from work, tired after a busy day caring for people. Imagine that you were asked what you had done that day, what you had worked on, what you had achieved. Your reply may be something like 'Well, loads of things. I don't know *what* exactly, but I know I have been really busy.' Now imagine that the whole of nursing is just like your day has been. Just like you, nursing does not really know what it has done or why; it knows only that it has been busy. Now ask yourself whether this image of nursing is one that would attract research funding. Medicine has a clear focus: we all know what it does - it tries to cure illness and make people better. Nursing does do some amazing things, but perhaps it needs to be clearer about what it does.

Other healthcare disciplines tend to be much 'smaller' than nursing, although they usually have a tighter professional focus; at least we 'know' what a physiotherapist does. Nevertheless, postgraduate activity in some of the smaller disciplines is still relatively under-developed. Perhaps it is when practitioners are doing masters and doctoral courses that they are most likely to begin to embark on research.

Nursing's professional status was, for a time, largely dependent on its association with medicine. In short, and for a variety of reasons, nursing did not freely embrace research but was content to conduct its practice based on custom and tradition (Walsh and Ford 1989a, b, c). In part, at least, nursing remains a little uncomfortable with research; there are no clearly visible funding streams for nursing research, and nursing is perhaps a little less clear than it ought to be about its central focus and purpose. All these factors militate against nursing practice being supported by research and other forms of evidence. However, things are changing and, although there is still much more that can be done in relation to research, nursing does now embrace the principle of evidence-based practice. Nursing is undergoing an evolutionary process in which research will play a central part. In addition, the move of nurse education into the university sector will gradually have the effect of empowering nurses to think about research, to use research and to conduct research themselves. It is clear that the other healthcare disciplines are also embracing evidence-based practice but that, as is the case in nursing, this is an evolutionary process.

Perhaps it is the case that the kind of evidence used to support and develop practice is less important than a willingness to use evidence. In the real world, and with resources that are often limited, it is sometimes necessary to accept evidence that is second best. This is true of all practice disciplines that deal with human beings. In the long run, however, what matters is a willingness to drive practice forward, to make things better and to expose new initiatives to one's peers so that those initiatives may be appropriately critiqued and so that others can learn from what we have managed to do. This energy, this wish to take responsibility for the development of our area of practice, is what marks out a profession from other occupational groups.

The ethics of research

The history of research in healthcare is replete with examples of imaginative and heroic endeavour. Medical researchers were often clinicians who indulged in research in their spare time. We owe much of what we know today to early research that was practised on patients' and (often) doctors' own bodies (Trumble and Cavanagh 2006; Grossman 2008). Although much has been learned from this research, rather too much harm has also been done. The early researchers of X-ray technology often succumbed to malignant disease secondary to the radiation inflicted on themselves in the hope of discovering more and more about the technology. Sometimes, doctors have been rather too keen to try out their new ideas on patients, who were not always kept fully informed about the dangers inherent in the new technique. Perhaps the worst example of this is that of lobotomy, where 'difficult' patients in mental health settings had their frontal lobe removed to cause them to become placid and compliant.

Example from the literature and research

Ken Kesey's book *One Flew Over the Cuckoo's Nest* is a novel about the way that lobotomy was used to control the behaviour of disruptive patients (Kesey 1962). The novel was made into a film by Milos Forman in 1975.

Example from practice

Charles Grossman (2008) describes the first use of penicillin in the USA. The drug was sent by post from England. When the doctors opened the package, they did not know what to do with the brown substance in the vial, there being no guidance on the matter. The doctors decided to dissolve the contents of the vial in saline and pass the resulting mixture through an asbestos filter in the hope of purifying it. The recipient of the drug was a moribund patient who was suffering from a fulminating infection. The patient survived.

It is sometimes difficult to separate clinical practice, which has as its aim the welfare of one particular patient, and clinical research, which chiefly aims to help future patients. However, there is an important distinction between the two. If you were to go into hospital for treatment, then you would expect that treatment to be wholly directed to your welfare and not compromised by any expectations that what can be learned from your case might help others. You may well be prepared to be the subject of an experiment, but you would expect to be made perfectly aware that that was what was going on. In practice, it is only too easy for a practitioner to 'just try something out' on a patient, but this is wrong on at least two counts: first, practice should be evidence-based and not 'evidence-generating'; and second, patients have a right to be treated as ill people and not as the subjects of an experiment.

Practitioners who carry out research need to regard their two roles as separate. Someone working as a staff nurse has access to patients' records. The nurse does not need permission to read a patient's notes. However, that same nurse, when working on his or her research project, has no right of access to patients' notes; for this, our nurse researcher must obtain consent from the patient and authority from the relevant ethics committee. The two roles of practitioner and researcher are separate, even when practised by the same person on the same day.

The importance of clinical research ethics was highlighted in the mid-twentieth century, when doctors (supported by nurses) working for the Nazi regime experimented on civilian prisoners (Lefor 2005). Such experiments included the use of surgery without anaesthesia and exposing people to extreme cold. These events remain today as evidence of the potential of medicine to cause deliberate harm in the name of research and science. In response to this, the Nuremberg Code (1949) and the Declaration of Helsinki (World Medical Association 1964; Williams 2008), adopted in 1964, established the core principles of research ethics. Today, the codes of research ethics published by each professional discipline (Royal College of Nursing 2007) exist to ensure that all planned research is ethically scrutinised.

The Royal College of Nursing (RCN) code of research ethics can be downloaded free of charge from the RCN website: www.rcn.org.uk/.

Principal considerations

- Research is an important way in which nursing and healthcare improve the quality of their provision.

- All research planning should be subject to oversight by the local research ethics committee and in healthcare by the system of research governance set up by the government (see the Department of Health website at www.dh.gov.uk).

- Research should be well designed and of good quality.

- The research should be justifiable in terms of potential benefits.

- Research should be safe, and any potential to cause harm should be considered in relation to the considered benefits of the research.

- The potential benefits of the research may not necessarily justify exposing participants to risk.

- There should be informed consent.

- Children and vulnerable people present special difficulties, principally in relation to informed consent. It may not always be ethically appropriate for parents and guardians to consent on behalf of children.

- Information about participants should be held confidentially and data should be secure.

- Participants have the right to withdraw at any time.

> Your own university will have a research ethics committee. Find out who is the chairperson, go and see them and ask if you can sit in on a committee meeting as an observer. This will be an interesting experience that will teach you a lot about the ways in which research proposals are scrutinised.

Published research will tend to mention research ethics only if ethical considerations have impacted on the design of the research. Often, the published paper will not even mention that ethical approval was given for the study to go ahead. However, one should not be concerned at this. Authors often have very little space in which to communicate their research to the readers and so ethical issues tend to be left out of the discussion. All clinical research and just about every other sort of research as well does have to be approved by the relevant research ethics committee, and it is reasonable to expect that this has been done.

Concluding remarks

In this chapter we have seen that research is not the only mechanism we have for producing new knowledge. In fact, there exists a wide range of other forms of evidence. We have noted, however, that research remains the gold standard and that we need to be careful before accepting other forms of evidence. We have seen that it is not always possible to undertake formal research on people, especially when they are vulnerable and unwell. Thus, we have to ensure that research complies with established ethical principles and guidelines, and so we often have to accept lower forms of evidence. This means that, in practice, the practitioner has always to bear in mind that we may not always know things as well as we think we do. It follows from this that the health care practitioner should take available opportunities to improve the quality of existing evidence, whether that means using such tools as audit or benchmarking or embarking on formal research.

Summary ──────────────────────────●

- It is a principle of evidence-based practice that the practitioner should always be able to defend their practice by identifying the degree to which it is supported by evidence.

- Well-designed research studies provide us with the best evidence with which to support and develop practice.

- Good-quality, well-designed research studies are expensive and may be ethically problematic in a discipline that deals with vulnerable people. For this reason, it is often necessary to have recourse to research designs that are less than perfect and to forms of non-research evidence.

- There are several forms of non-research evidence that can be used usefully to support and develop practice. These include such techniques as peer review, exposing ideas to publication and benchmarking.

- Care should be taken in accepting all forms of evidence. Each should be examined logically. Non-research forms of evidence are particularly vulnerable to human error, to bias and to the effect of variables that may be unidentified or poorly understood.

- Of central importance is the practitioner's enthusiasm for practice and the desire to make things better. Practice should be founded in evidence, and practitioners who are enthusiastic about their work will want to use evidence to support and to develop practice for the good of patients and for the good of the whole profession.

- All research must comply with ethical standards and be approved by the local research ethics committee and, in the NHS, by the system of research governance set up by the government. Practical guidance on research ethics are published by the various healthcare professions, including the RCN.

Further reading

This paper looks at the use of peer review (peer observation):

Davys, D. and V. Jones (2007). 'Peer observation: a tool for continuing professional development . . . including commentaries by Dominique Lowenthal and Dr. Joanna Jackson'. *International Journal of Therapy and Rehabilitation* **14**(11): 489–493.

This paper discusses the difficulties involved in basing practice upon evidence rather than conventional wisdom. The authors conclude that evidence-based practice is really the only way to go, despite the difficulties:

Herbert, R. D., C. Sherrington, C. Maher and A. M. Moseley (2001). 'Evidence-based practice – imperfect but necessary'. *Physiotherapy Theory and Practice* **17**(3): 201–211.

Here is a paper that looks at the way in which benchmarking can be used to improve practice:

Neill, C. and U. Hughes (2004). 'Improving inter-hospital transfer'. *Paediatric Nursing* **16**(7): 24–27.

This is the reference for the RCN guidance on research ethics:

Royal College of Nursing (2007). *Research Ethics: RCN Guidance for Nurses.* London: Royal College of Nursing.

This paper discusses the ways in which clinical guidelines can be developed through the use of clinical governance:

Stewart, E. (2006). 'Nursing guidelines: development of catheter care guidelines for Guy's and St Thomas''. *British Journal of Nursing (BJN)* **15**(8): 420.

This paper considers peer review:

Yoder-Wise, P. S. (2008). 'The value of peer review: the hard workers behind the scenes'. *Journal of Continuing Education in Nursing* **39**(4): 147–148.

References

Castledine, G. (2008). 'Overzealousness in accident and emergency nursing'. *British Journal of Nursing (BJN)* **17**(18): 1199.

Duncombe, M. A. (1979). *A Brief History of the Association of British Paediatric Nurses 1938-1975.* London: Association of British Paediatric Nurses.

Dyer, I. (1997). 'The significance of statistical significance'. *Intensive and Critical Care Nursing* **13**(5): 259–265.

Gordon, M. (1994). *Nursing Diagnosis, Process and Applications*. St Louis, IL: Mosby.

Grossman, C. M. (2008). 'History of medicine: the first use of penicillin in the United States'. *Annals of Internal Medicine* **149**(2): 135-136.

Herbert, R. D., C. Sherrington, C. Maher and A. M. Moseley (2001). 'Evidence-based practice: imperfect but necessary'. *Physiotherapy Theory and Practice* **17**(3): 201-211.

Jolley, J. (2007). 'Separation and psychological trauma: a paradox examined'. *Paediatric Nursing* **19**(3): 22-25.

Jolley, J. (2008). 'The enlightened sixties'. *Paediatric Nursing* **20**(2): 12.

Jolley, J. and L. Shields (2009). 'The evolution of family-centered care'. *Journal of Pediatric Nursing* **24**(2): 164-170.

Kesey, K. (1962). *One Flew Over the Cuckoo's Nest*. New York: Viking Press.

Lefor, A. T. (2005). 'Scientific misconduct and unethical human experimentation: historic parallels and moral implications'. *Nutrition* **21**(7/8): 878-882.

Murphy, F. (2006). 'Dialysis: a care study exploring a patient's non-compliance to haemodialysis'. *British Journal of Nursing (BJN)* **15**(14): 773-776.

Nuremberg Code (1949). *Trials of War Criminals before the Nuremberg Military Tribunals under Control Council Law*. Washington, DC: US Government Printing Office.

Royal College of Nursing (2007). *Research Ethics: RCN Guidance for Nurses*. London: Royal College of Nursing.

Stewart, E. (2006). 'Nursing guidelines: development of catheter care guidelines for Guy's and St Thomas''. *British Journal of Nursing (BJN)* **15**(8): 420.

Trumble, S. and K. Cavanagh (2006). 'Shades of grey'. *Australian Family Physician* **35**(5): 277.

Walsh, M. and P. Ford (1989a). *Nursing Rituals, Research and Rational Actions*. London, Heinemann.

Walsh, M. and P. Ford (1989b). 'Rituals in nursing: "we always do it this way" . . . part 1'. *Nursing Times* **85**(41): 26.

Walsh, M. and P. Ford (1989c). 'We always do it this way: rituals in nursing in the surgical area examined in the light of research based evidence'. *Nursing Times and Nursing Mirror* **85**: 26-35.

Williams, J. R. (2008). 'The Declaration of Helsinki and public health . . . original declaration reproduced in full with permission of the World Medical Association'. *Bulletin of the World Health Organization* **86**(8): 650–652.

World Medical Association (1964). *Declaration of Helsinki*. Helsinki: World Medical Association.

Xu, W., A. D. Towers, P. Li and J. Collet (2006). 'Traditional Chinese medicine in cancer care: perspectives and experiences of patients and professionals in China'. *European Journal of Cancer Care* **15**(4): 397–403.

Chapter 4
Research methods and design

CHAPTER OBJECTIVES

The objectives for this chapter are to:

- Discuss the need for research studies to be well planned and fit for purpose

- Identify those methodologies that are commonly used in healthcare research.

Chapter outline

This chapter is about how research is planned and designed.

By now you will have developed an understanding in your own mind about how research fits with clinical practice. We should be ready for the next challenge: to make sense of some of the most commonly used kinds of research design.

You have already come across the two most important kinds of research: quantitative and qualitative research. Now we will look more closely, particularly at quantitative research, to identify some of the more important subtypes of research. It is not necessary to know about every kind of research design, but knowing some of the more important ones will be a great beginning and will allow you to make sense of other research methodologies as and when you come across them.

Design and method

Anything good needs to be well planned. Research often requires the invest-ment of a considerable amount of time, and no one wants to waste their time on a badly conceived project. In this, research is just like any other project: it is just like planning to build a new house, for example. Get your house design wrong and you could waste a lot of time and money.

If you do wish to build your own house, you will need to spend some time planning the build. Houses don't just spring up by themselves. More than this, you might want the house to be just right for you and your family, especially if you are spending a lot of time and money on the venture. Building your new house will be quite a project for you and that is exactly what it will be – a project. You will need to design the house. You might want to build a modern house with all the latest labour-saving and energy-efficient gadgets. On the other hand, you might want to build a more traditional-looking house with an emphasis on good-quality materials and that looks fabulous. If you have sufficient funds, you can design the house of your dreams, as long as the design is good. It wouldn't do to build a house that was beautiful but that fell down during the first winter storm. There is more than one possible design but, whatever the design is, it needs to be good and fit for the purpose for which it is intended. In the same way, research needs to be designed, it needs to be planned; there are many available designs, but whichever is used, it needs to be good. Sometimes, researchers substitute the word 'robust' for 'good'. A research design should be robust. That is, it should be fit for purpose, just like your house, and it should withstand any criticism, just like your house needs to withstand the winter storms.

You can build your house using one of several available methods. After the Second World War people built lots of prefabricated houses because they needed to build houses quickly (Stevenson 2003). You might wish to have your house hand-crafted from the best wood or you might choose to use bricks or concrete. You will build your house using the method of your choice. In the same way, research studies all employ a method; in other words, the design of the study is implemented, or carried out, using a method.

So, the design of a study is 'what will be done' and the method of a study is 'how it will be done'. When you plan your new house, you will probably plan the design and the method of building at more or less the same time. In fact, that is a good idea. It is just the same with research; indeed, people often use the form 'design and method' together. Sometimes, they like to sound important, so they use the words 'design and methodology'; this sounds much more intellectual. However, we all now know that it means nothing more than the way the research is planned – that is, its design and the methods that are to be used to implement that design. The design and methodology exist as the plan for the research, a kind of road map of how the research will be executed. The plan is like the instructions that you will give the builders so that they can build your new house to your exact specifications.

If you are thinking of purchasing an existing house, you will want to know about its structure and how it was built. The same is true of research: the design and methodology of any study are of interest to those who may wish to critique the study. It is important that the design and methodology of the research are available because, unlike a house, which anyone can see, it isn't always possible to tell from data how those data were collected. So, design and methodology are about the planning of research. However, the design and methodology of a study are just as important *after* the study is completed because they allow others to judge the quality of the study.

The elements of research design

There are a range of things that need to be considered when planning any research. These fall conveniently into the following categories.

- *Quantitative or qualitative*: quantitative research tries to identify the facts about something, whereas qualitative research tries to explore and find meaning in something. Usually, quantitative research deals with numbers whereas qualitative research deals with verbal or textual material.

- *Descriptive, experimental and explorative*: descriptive research tries to identify 'what is' or 'what has been'. Experimental research (experiments) is concerned with 'what if' situations to develop new ways of doing things. Explorative research is often qualitative and aims to provide a new insight into things. Sometimes, this is a first step to other forms of research but at other times it is sufficient in itself.

- *The amount of control*: control is arguably more of an issue for quantitative research. The researcher has to make decisions about the degree to which sampling, random allocation and blinding are used.

- *The design*: it may be necessary to have only one group within which data are collected. A survey often has only one body (group) of data. However, an experiment may involve having a control group; for example, for reasons of comparison. Designs can be very simple (one group) or they can be quite complex.

New words

Sampling It is not always possible to collect data from everything or every person in which we are interested. In this situation, the researcher will some-times collect data only from a sample. In this case, steps need to be taken to ensure that the sample is representative of the whole (the population).

Random allocation This is the process by which the researcher ensures that each participant has an equal chance of being selected in the study and allocated to a group (for example, the experimental group or the control group) within the study. It is a way in which an attempt is made to reduce the possibility of bias.

Blinding This is not as brutal as it sounds. Blinding is the process of ensuring that the individuals who provide, collect and interpret the data do not know which group they are in. For example, a patient in a drug trial might not know whether they have been taking the drug or a placebo, and a researcher collecting data from patients might not know whether each patient (participant) has been exposed to the treatment or is in the control group. Blinding is another means of reducing the possibility of bias or the unconscious interpretation of data.

Most of this is just common sense. It can seem complicated because there are a lot of ways in which research can be conducted. We need to have labels for all of these methods to communicate them. None of these research methods is difficult to understand; it is just that there are a lot of them. In addition, not all the terms are mutually exclusive; in this way, we can have qualitative descriptive studies but we can also have quantitative descriptive studies. Nevertheless, designing a research study is so common-sense that you could design one now. The section below presents a research problem and asks you to design a suitable study. You will be given prompts so that all you need to do is tick a few boxes. So, let's see whether you can design your own research project.

Design your own study

This study is concerned with the choices made by nursing students at the end of their first year of study. You need to find out how many of them think that they have selected the right field (adult nursing, children's nursing, mental health nursing, learning disability nursing) and how many think that they would like to reconsider their area of specialism. You don't need to explore their feelings on the matter; rather, you simply want to know whether they are happy with their choice or whether they may decide to change to another field.

Now design a study that would be most appropriate. Here are some prompts – just tick the boxes.

Is the study quantitative or qualitative?

Quantitative research tries to identify the facts about something, whereas qualitative research tries to explore and find meaning in something. Usually, quantitative research deals with numbers whereas qualitative research deals with verbal or textual material.

Quantitative ☐

Qualitative ☐

Is the study descriptive, experimental or explorative?

Descriptive research tries to identify 'what is' or 'what has been'. Experimental research (experiments) is concerned with 'what if' situations to develop new ways of doing things. Explorative research is often qualitative and aims to provide a new insight into things. Sometimes this is a first step to other forms of research, but at other times it is sufficient in itself.

Descriptive ☐

Experimental ☐

Explorative ☐

Will you take a sample or use all of the end-of-first-year students?

Take a sample ☐

Use all of the students ☐

What design will you use?

It may be necessary only to have one group within which data are collected. A survey often has only one body of data. However, an experiment may involve having a control group; for example, for reasons of comparison. Designs can be very simple (one group) or quite complex.

One group ☐

Two or more groups to enable a control ☐

What controls will you design into the research?

Control is arguably more of an issue for quantitative research. The researcher has to make decisions about the degree to which sampling, random allocation and blinding are used.

Will you use randomisation (for selection and allocation to groups)?

Randomisation for selection (if used) of students ☐

Randomisation for the placement of students into experimental and control groups (if used) ☐

No randomisation ☐

Blinding – will you keep any aspect of the research secret from the participants (students) or the people collecting or interpreting the data?

Blinding of participants (so they don't know which group they are in) ☐

Blinding of data collectors or those interpreting the data (so they don't know which group the participants are in) ☐

No blinding ☐

So, how did you design your study? Here are the appropriate answers:

Quantitative or qualitative?

Quantitative   ☑

Qualitative   ☐

We are collecting data about people's choices. We can do this quantitatively because we do not want to ask the students about their motivation or feelings about which branch to move to.

Descriptive, experimental or explorative?

Descriptive   ☑

Experimental   ☐

Explorative   ☐

This is a descriptive study: it is describing 'what is'. The students have made their decision (or have decided that they are unsure) and we simply need to find out what it is they have decided.

Use a sample or use all of the end-of-first-year students?

Take a sample   ☐

Use all of the students   ☑

We could take a sample here, but we probably want to know what each actual student wants to do.

Which design?

One group   ☑

Two or more groups to enable a control   ☐

We need only one group of students. We don't have a group for each branch. We have one group of students who will tell us which branch they wish to enter. We don't need a control group, because there is nothing to control.

Randomisation?

Randomisation for selection of students ☐

Randomisation for the placement of students into experimental
and control groups ☐

No randomisation ☑

*There is only one group of students and we have used the whole cohort –
so randomisation is not needed.*

Blinding?

Blinding of participants (so they don't know which group they are in) ☐

Blinding of data collectors or those interpreting the data
(so they don't know which group the participants are in) ☐

No blinding ☑

*There is only one group of students. The students can't be blinded because
they already know who they are. As there is no control group, blinding
cannot be used in relation to the researchers' knowledge of which students
are in which group.*

The chances are that you either made the same decisions as those listed
above *or* you have good reason for making other decisions. Perhaps you chose
a qualitative study because you wanted to explore the students' thinking
behind their choice of branch. Indeed, this might make a very interesting
study. You may have chosen to use a sample. This might be a good idea if
we were interested in generalities, such as the likelihood that more students
are going to want to change branch this year compared with last year. Sampling
may also be necessary if the population of students (that is, all of them) is
very large.

So, you have just designed your first research study. You did it with common
sense, intelligence and analysis. Whatever we know about research, whatever
experience we have, it is most important that we use those very same qualities
when designing a study. Knowledge is never enough. The most experienced
researcher needs the skills that you have just employed here.

Types of design

One of the reasons that research can seem complicated is the multiplicity of available designs. House building is complicated in the same way: there are just so many designs for houses. Questions inevitably arise as to which design is best, most fit for purpose, most robust, etc. It is not necessary to learn about all the research designs ever conceived. Most professional researchers are familiar with just a few designs that are relevant to their area of research, so it would be unfair to expect you to know more than they do. Rather, it is better for you to learn just one or two designs. Learn these well and they will provide a good foundation for a solid understanding of research. In time you may come across other designs, but these will make more sense, more easily, because you will be able to compare them with the one or two designs you learn now.

Research designs, just like the design of a house, are logical and systematic; they are plain, black-and-white, straight-talking things. You wouldn't want any 'grey' areas in your house design, any places where questions could arise about what exactly you wanted. In the same way, the research design is a deeply practical thing. The design is logically contrived; this means (just about) that it is drawn up using a lot of common sense and a little bit of knowledge.

We have already seen that you could design your own research study, just by using your common sense. However, there are a few kinds of research design of which you need to be aware. Most research will be planned using one of the designs below.

- *Qualitative*: usually purposed to 'explore' a phenomenon

- *Quantitative*: there are two main groups of quantitative designs:

  - *Descriptive* (or 'non-experiment'), identifying 'what is' situations. Sometimes descriptive studies have just one group of data, and sometimes there is more than one group so that differences can be identified. However, descriptive studies are retrospective; they measure 'what is' (what has been).
  - *Experimental*, identifying 'what if' situations. These are sometimes called prospective designs because they are producing situations that do not exist at the moment.

We should be clear that there is more than one way to design studies that use one of these main design groupings. However, it is far more important to understand the difference between an experiment and a non-experiment, for example, than it is to understand the several different forms an experiment can take. There is not a 'best' design, although some designs do tend to suit some disciplines and some situations. Medicine tends to use the experimental design whereas sociology tends to use surveys and descriptive studies. Nursing is an eclectic discipline and, as such, uses a wide range of designs. This does make it really quite difficult to get a grasp on nursing research overall. Doctors are much luckier: once they have understood a randomised control trial, they will have learned all they need to know about research. Nurses, on the other hand, have a much harder time of it: there is barely any type of research design that is not used in nursing.

Deductive and inductive research

To deduce something is to reach a conclusion about a question by drawing on one or more general principles. We may, for example, attempt to explain an adolescent's behaviour by using Piagetian theory of human development (Piaget 1952; Piaget and Inhelder 1972). Researchers sometimes do the same thing with their research; they allow existing theory to guide the research (see Fincham and Jaspars 1979). Deductive research is more commonly found in disciplines that have well-developed theories. If you were to ask a psychologist to explain their work, they might say that they were a Freudian psychologist, a cognitive psychologist or a behavioural psychologist. These terms represent major theoretical streams of thought (theories). It is not surprising, then, that a behavioural psychologist might want behaviourist theory to guide each stage of the research process. Researchers are explicit about the theory that has underpinned their research and sometimes write a section of their research report on the theoretical underpinning or the theoretical model that has been used.

Students are sometimes asked to plan a potential research study. On occasions, they are asked to include a chapter on the theoretical model that has been used to guide the research.

This is all very unfortunate because most healthcare students will find that they can't think of any theories and those they do know about simply don't seem to fit their proposal.

This comes about because some people think that healthcare should have lots of theories. Psychology and sociology have theories, so healthcare practitioners should have some too. However, the healthcare disciplines are not psychology, but are practice disciplines that deal with facts about practice rather than theories about the universe.

Deductive research is not so commonly found in the healthcare disciplines, such as nursing. Nursing is rightly a pragmatic and practice-focused discipline. It uses a unique mix of knowledge from many different disciplines and arguably does not have theories of its own. If you asked a nurse to explain their work, they might tell you what sort of ward they worked on but it is unlikely that they would explain their work by making reference to a nursing theory. We should not worry about this; it doesn't make us any less clever or any less academic. In fact, medicine is in much the same position; there are no real theories of medicine. Medicine, too, simply uses a unique mix of knowledge from other disciplines such as pharmacology, histology and even nursing. What differentiates medicine from nursing is that the two disciplines use a different mix of knowledge.

Nursing and medicine tend to use inductive research (see Maputle and Nolte 2008). To reason inductively is to draw general principles from detail. In this way, we might look at an adolescent's behaviour and come to a new under-standing of adolescence, which we might then use to help us to understand the behaviour of other adolescents. Inductive research is a bottom-up approach: it deals with questions about the particular (about practice) and aims to create a new understanding. Indeed, inductive research is often the way in which theory is developed. Healthcare practitioners and doctors tend to be interested in details about practice. They ask questions such as 'How can we better control procedural pain?' and 'Why do these children appear to be so afraid of injections?' Research into the former may eventually help us to better under-stand pain itself (we will be developing a new theory of pain). In the second example, research into children's fear of injections may in time help us to understand the way that children construe invasive techniques.

New words

Variable Something that varies. A variable can be the thing that is being observed and tested in research. In an experiment, the *independent variable* is the treatment, the thing that is designed to cause an effect on the dependent variable. The *dependent variable* is the thing that reacts to being experimented on. It is the thing in which the effect of the intervention is witnessed and measured.

Qualitative designs

The term 'qualitative' is a little misleading because quantitative methodologies are often employed to look at the quality of something. It is better to consider qualitative methodologies as those that explore feelings, personal inter- pretations and experiences. It follows that qualitative studies only ever involve people (not planets, motor cars or animals). Also, it is usually the case that qualitative studies collect verbal or written data rather than numbers. This is simply because feelings, personal interpretations and experiences are usually best explored using language rather than numbers. The key here is 'explora- tion'. We could ask someone to rate their level of happiness on a 5-point scale but to explore their perception of happiness using a numerical scale would be difficult. So it is that qualitative studies are associated with some kind of verbal dialogue between the researcher and the participant.

The purpose of qualitative studies tends to be different from that of quantit- ative studies. In the former, the researcher usually wants to know about one or more people and there is little, if any, attempt to argue for these people being representative of a population. It is because of this that it is sometimes said that qualitative studies are rather less scientific than quantitative studies. In addition, qualitative studies usually fail the normal criteria for robustness that are applied to quantitative studies. There is no random allocation, no blinding and no means to ensure accurate sampling. However, such concern is mis- guided, for research is simply a systematic enquiry, and qualitative studies are both an enquiry and systematic. Qualitative studies are logically determined (well planned) and are focused. Furthermore, qualitative studies address important areas of human existence that could simply not be addressed by quantitative research.

In the past, you will probably have been given a questionnaire like this one:

Module evaluation

How would you rate the module overall?

Poor   ☐
Average   ☐
Good   ☐

Perhaps you look at this and think, 'Well, it was somewhere between average and good.' Perhaps you look at it and say 'But what *is* average? What *is* good? While you can respond to questions like this, you probably value the opportunity to discuss the module with the teaching staff. Such a discussion is more likely to enable you to express just exactly how you feel about the module. The question above is essentially quantitative; the discussion you have with the module leader is essentially qualitative.

Healthcare practice deals with many issues that are better communicated using the rich language that we all possess. In this way, qualitative research often deals with people's experiences that are sensitive, emotive and valuable. It would often be inappropriate to try to put these experiences into prelabelled boxes – and if we did such a thing, we would get a very distorted view of reality.

Qualitative studies are just as focused as any other kind of research. These studies clearly identify the research problem (the focus of the research) and the way in which participants were selected. However, qualitative studies do not usually deal with a sample because there is no population to be sampled. This is because most qualitative studies do not claim that their data are representative of that which might be obtained from other people. In any case, the number of participants (the sample size) tends to be quite small, often fewer than 10 people. Such studies are a systematic enquiry into those 10 people. Nevertheless, it is important to recruit participants carefully. If the research is focused on patients' experience of pain management, then there would be little point in recruiting patients who had not experienced pain. Because qualitative studies often focus on difficult and traumatic experiences, the search for and recruitment of suitable participants can be a protracted process and one that requires a professionally mature and sensitive approach.

The number of participants recruited in the study is often determined by data saturation. This means that when one begins to obtain the same information from subsequent participants, there is little point in continuing with the data collection. At this point, the data are said to be 'saturated' and the recruitment of new participants is stopped.

There are no experimental and control groups in qualitative studies. Usually, there is just one group of participants, although sometimes two or more groups can be established when a degree of comparison is warranted. Most qualitative studies, however, have only one group of participants.

Most planning decisions for qualitative studies relate to how participants will be questioned. For example, it may be better to interview participants one at a time or to enable a group of participants to discuss questions together (a focus group). It may be necessary to conduct only one interview or several interviews, many may even be needed. As always, the planning for this should be based on what makes most sense in relation to what the research is goaled to explore.

It is the case with almost any research that the researcher hopes to summarise the data and to make the data understandable. In quantitative studies, the researcher might use statistical analysis, which in part works to provide a suc-cinct summary of the data. In just the same way, the qualitative researcher will try to summarise what often amounts to many hours of interview data. In most cases, a form of content analysis is used to create themes or commonalities in the data. These themes may then be presented to the participants as a way of asking them 'Does this summarise what you told me?' Sometimes, the participants will respond, 'Well, no, not really' or 'Well, partly', in which case the researcher will have to do some work on the themes until the participants are happy that they reflect what they said in the interviews. Perhaps you can see that the data collection and the analysis can become merged into one process in qualitative research. This is because the process of providing the data is a learned experience. Participants' understanding of what they have experienced (the focus of the research) can and often does change as they go through the process of communicating that experience. The researcher, too, often becomes part of this process. There is at least a sharing of responsibility for the data between the researcher and the participants, with all parties being committed to producing information that accurately reflects what has been and is being experienced. Much of the planning for qualitative research is focused on these aspects of the study, namely the collection, re-collection and ongoing analysis of the data.

Some common types of qualitative research

Qualitative research will be discussed in more detail in subsequent chapters. However, it is useful here just to note the most common forms of qualitative research.

Phenomenology

Phenomenology attempts to describe individuals' lived experiences. Phenom-enology can look to the outsider as if it deals with the subjective world. However, phenomenologists take the view that what people perceive as real is in fact real and therefore objective to that person. Phenomenology seeks to identify the meanings that people find in their experience; for example, of being hospitalised or of giving birth. It is necessary for this meaning to be shared with the researcher, and thus a common understanding is reached.

Example from the literature and research

In a phenomenological study, Rosedale (2009) found that women who had survived breast cancer felt lonely and isolated but that at the same time they developed a deeper relationship with their children and found themselves to be more compassionate and understanding of the suffering of others. The phenomenological orientation of the research study helped to focus the research on the way in which the women found meaning in the way their relationship with others had changed.

Grounded theory research

Grounded theory was developed by Glaser and Strauss (1967) and is inductive in nature, immersing itself in the personal realities of human experience. Grounded theory research is used where no previous research exists. In this way, grounded theory research is used to explore new areas of human experience. Grounded theory does not use existing theoretical frameworks but aims to generate a new theory of the aspect of human experience being examined.

Ethnographical research

Ethnographical research developed from anthropology. Ethno means 'people' (as in 'ethnic') and graphic means 'drawing' or 'picture'. Ethnographic research focuses on culture (a particular culture or an aspect of culture) and examines people's behaviour within that culture or the differences between two cultures. Just like anthropologists, ethnographical researchers will immerse themselves in the culture being examined and will seek to become accepted by the people they wish to study. The researcher will then identify participants who are willing to talk about the aspects of their lives that are central to the culture in question. Ethnographic research concerns itself with such diverse cultures as those of remote tribes or that of nursing in the UK.

Qualitative research can be particularly interesting and does have the advantage (for some) that it rarely involves any statistical analysis. The output of qualitative research can be easier to understand than that of quantitative research. In many ways, qualitative research seems to suit the healthcare professions, which, after all, have a focus on care and on human experience.

> ## Example from the literature and research
>
> Using an ethnographical approach, Roberts (2008) worked within the culture of nursing to examine the ways in which student nurses helped each other to learn. The research found that students formed friendships with other students and that these friendship groups were used to provide peer support for learning.

Quantitative designs

In some ways, quantitative designs seem harder to understand than qualitative designs because there are so many of them. For this reason, we need not worry about identifying every type of design. Instead, let's look at the main forms that quantitative designs take. You will gradually learn about new designs as you read more about research and as you begin to put this into practice.

The survey

A survey has a single group of participants, such as a sample of people eligible to vote at the next election. A survey is also descriptive; it aims to describe one or more aspects of the sample. For example, a survey may aim to describe how people claim they intend to vote at the next election. A survey is not an experiment because there is no independent variable. Our survey would become an experiment only if, for example, we showed one group of participants a film (the independent variable) of how poor university students had become, before asking them how they might vote at the next election. We might then compare the results from this group with those from a control group who had not been shown the film about impoverished university students.

A survey may be simple, but sometimes it is exactly the right choice. At some point, you will have been asked to evaluate a module or course of study at your university. In this case, the university simply wants to know what its students think of the course; it wants to use standard questions with closed, multiple-choice-like responses. For this, a survey is both simple and perfect.

Module evaluation

How would you rate the module overall?

Poor ☐
Average ☐
Good ☐

New words

Differences and correlations Often we want to consider the difference between one set of data and another set of data, and most statistical procedures are designed to do this. Sometimes, however, we want to determine the degree to which one set of data agrees with or matches another. For example, as children grow older, they tend to grow taller; indeed, age and height in childhood do correlate positively.

The survey design is so simple that you might wonder why one should ever use anything more complicated. However, on the whole, we can only analyse survey data descriptively. This means that we can calculate descriptive statistics such as counts and percentages but we cannot easily determine differences or correlations between two groups of data. So, a survey is good for describing what is, usually from one group of data. If this is what we want to do and we are sure we won't want to do anything else, then a survey is perfect.

Although a survey usually has only one group of data, it is sometimes possible to split the data into two or more groups. For example, a survey of potential voting behaviour could look for the existence of differences between male and female voters. This may be reasonable where we are simply attempting to describe 'what is' in relation to the sample as a whole. However, we may quickly run into problems with the sample size for males and females if we do not select the sample with a view to studying the variable of gender. Also, we would really need to ensure that the sampling procedure we used was capable of selecting an unbiased sample of both men and (separately) women. In practice, it would be a good idea to have deliberately set out to study the voting patterns of men and women, rather than to decide to do so after we have generated the data.

Planning is important. Of course you could design and build your house with three bedrooms and then decide to add another bedroom later. However, people will always know that that room was added later; you will never get the colour and style of brick to match that used in the rest of the house. It is just like that with research. It is rarely possible to get away with bad planning. If we want to look at the voting behaviour of men and women and how men and women vote differently (if they do), then we should design our research for this purpose – and if we did, we would probably choose not to use a survey.

The descriptive design

The word 'descriptive' is used here largely for want of a better word. However, what we mean here is a design that is not a survey because it has more than one group designed into it but it is not an experiment because it seeks only to describe 'what is'. A descriptive design does not have an independent variable because it is not seeking to test out something new. Some people call this sort of design 'retrospective'; this is another label meant to indicate that such studies aim to look at 'what is' (or, really, 'what has just been') situations. Descriptive research does not manipulate situations to study them; experiments do.

Descriptive studies lack some of the controls that can be put in place for experiments (prospective designs). In this way, there is no randomised control study for the descriptive design. It is not usually possible to have such controls in a situation where the researcher is studying what is already taking place. Perhaps, for example, we wish to look at two different nursing procedures in respect of how much pain they may cause. In this situation, the nursing pro-cedures have been practised for some time. It isn't possible to set up a control because all of the patients in this situation simply have to have one procedure or the other. However, some controls can be put in place. We may be able to provide a degree of randomisation in relation to the selection of participants and the allocation of them to groups. We could ensure that the person collect-ing the data is not aware of which procedure the patient had (blinding). Perhaps we could even ensure that the patient didn't know which procedure he or she had. In practice, however, these controls can be very difficult to apply to descriptive studies. It is a little like us having built our house, only then to decide that it would be good to put in an environmental monitoring facility to measure how energy-efficient the house is. We could probably do this, but it would certainly have been easier to have planned this into the design of the house from the beginning. The descriptive design is used where 'the house' is already built. That is the situation with which we are dealing; we can't undo the fact that 'the house' is already built.

There may be a tendency to criticise descriptive designs for the lack of control they are able to apply. However, randomisation, blinding and control groups may all be quite impossible to apply here. In practice, few, if any, research studies that involve human participants can ever be perfect. It is perhaps important only to make each study as robust as possible. The material that descriptive studies concern themselves with is the 'what is' situations of life as they are being played out today. It is often important that we research what happens today in clinical practice. Such studies sometimes lead in time to further experimental studies that can offer better control and that can develop new practices for the future.

The experimental design

We are all familiar with the notion of an experiment. It conjures up images of white-coated scientists messing about with test tubes over a Bunsen burner. This is actually a rather useful image because it is in the laboratory that experiments are most easily undertaken.

New words

Control group A group exposed to no treatment at all to determine what effect the treatment has.

Experiment Formally, an experiment is said to exist where the researcher introduces one or more independent variables to determine their effect on one or more dependent variables. However, the experimental design is also associated with studies that require a high level of control and with measures designed to ensure objectivity and freedom from bias.

Retrospective Relating to a descriptive design. The opposite is prospective, a term used for experiments.

In the laboratory, it is possible to have control over everything that happens. We can put mixture *a* into test tube *b* and do whatever we want with it. So, a high degree of control is one of the factors that characterise an experiment. It is not usually possible to acquire the same level of control when doing research with people.

The other main characteristic is that an experiment is dealing with novel situations. The researcher will be asking 'what if' questions such as 'What will happen if I mix substance *a* with substance *b*?' So, an experiment is associated with a high degree of control and it deals with new situations. An experiment is trying to discover things about future possibilities; in other words, it is prospective.

It is one thing to run an experiment in a laboratory but quite another to experiment with people. Healthcare practitioners tend to be interested in people more than in the content of test tubes. Human beings are difficult to control. We can imagine all kinds of interesting experiments with people, but the people concerned may not be prepared to be experimented on or may have views about their role within the experiment. Another major issue with experiments on people is that people are inherently variable. They change from day to day and from moment to moment. The laboratory scientist can control all or most of the variables so that they vary only when he or she wants them to; this is rarely possible when working with people. For this reason, experiments with people are rarely perfect.

New words

Randomised control trial A form of experimental design characterised by a high degree of control of the variables and of the data. As the name suggests, a randomised control trial (often abbreviated to RCT) will employ random allocation and at least one experimental and one control group.

Experimental or independent variable In experiments (quantitative studies), the experimental or independent variable is the thing that is thought to affect another variable. So, for example, if we measure the effect of giving or not giving a drug for pain, the giving or not giving the drug would be the experimental or independent variable. The resulting pain level would be the dependent variable.

Medicine often uses experimental designs. However, medicine's experiments most often involve drug trials. Here, variables are relatively easy to control. It is probably fair to say that, outside drug trials, medicine has the same problem with experiments as do the other healthcare disciplines.

Examples of research designs

Let us look at the variety of designs available in quantitative studies. We will start with the simplest designs and gradually begin to look at some more complex ones. The more complex designs often offer better control and are therefore more robust. However, bear in mind that sometimes a more simple design may be perfectly appropriate. If there were a best design, then everyone would use it and we would have to learn only that one design. When planning research, it is important to use the most appropriate design, and that often means using a simple one.

In Figure 4.1, there is just one group. Let's assume that this is a group of people who have been exposed to a nursing procedure associated with pain.

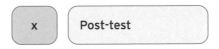

Figure 4.1 Research design for a single group.

There may be a lot that we want to find out about these people and their pain. However, let's assume that for the moment we simply want to find out how much pain these people are experiencing after they have been exposed to the nursing procedure in question.

So, this is our design. The $\boxed{x}$ stands for treatment, which is research language for the intervention to which the research participants are exposed. In this case, it is the nursing procedure that we think may be associated with pain.

The $\boxed{\text{Post-test}}$ box signifies the collection of data. Perhaps the research will involve the administration of a questionnaire that asks the participants to rate their pain on a scale of 1–10. The term 'post-test' is used to indicate that this comes after ('post') the intervention (nursing procedure) and that it is a 'test', meaning a collection of data.

This design is similar to that of a survey. First of all, it is descriptive; this is not an experiment. The reason that it is not an experiment is that we are measuring only what is already there. We are not introducing a new variable. Second, we have only one group of participants. However, we have selected participants who have had or who are having the nursing procedure in question. Surveys often use selection procedures, which can be quite focused and sophisticated. After all, there is no point in asking babies how they will vote at the next election.

Let's remind ourselves of what this study aimed to achieve – a measure of the amount of pain experienced by people who were exposed to the nursing procedure. This simple design should be sufficient. However, there are some things that this design would *not* enable the researcher to do. Think about it now and list below some limitations of this design. You don't need to know the answer to this question; you can use reason and analysis to work it out.

....

....

....

This design will not enable us to work out:

- whether these participants had pain before the procedure;
- whether their pain before the procedure was the same as the pain after the procedure;
- whether the pain was made better or made worse by the procedure.

However, this is not a problem, because the design was intended only to enable the study to determine the amount of perceived pain experienced by the participants after they had been exposed to the nursing procedure. Simple designs can be used to achieve simple outcomes. Indeed, it would be wasteful of resources to enable a design that would tell us more than we needed to know.

More complex designs

Let's look at that list above again:

- whether these participants had pain before the procedure;
- whether their pain before the procedure was the same as the pain after the procedure;
- whether the pain was made better or made worse by the procedure.

It is often the case that we want to find out whether an intervention makes a difference. Clearly, we could do this by adding a pre-test group. If we test the sample for pain before and after the intervention, then we will be able to determine what effect the intervention has had on the participants' pain (Figure 4.2).

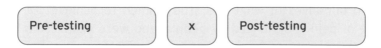

Figure 4.2 Research design using a pre- and post-test group.

Remember, *X* is the intervention, the effect of which we are examining. Exposure to *X* (the nursing intervention) is the independent variable. The participants' perceived pain is the dependent variable. So, this should do it. Now we are testing the participants' pain both before and after the intervention (a nursing procedure). This should enable us to determine the effect on perceived pain of the intervention. This is sometimes called a 'pre-test–post-test' design. This design may be perfectly adequate. It will tell us:

- whether these participants had pain before the procedure;

- whether their pain before the procedure was the same as the pain after the procedure;

- whether the pain was made better or made worse by the procedure.

But, research needs to be robust and resistant to criticism. Take another look at our pre-test–post-test design and see whether you can see a potential flaw in it.

We know that pain can be remedied by a wide range of things. We know that anxiety can increase pain and that reassurance can reduce pain (Oshodi 2007). Perhaps it is possible that the pre-testing might have the effect of reassuring the participants that they are cared about. After all, they haven't even had the procedure yet and someone is already asking them whether they have any pain. The mere presence of someone spending time with the participant and asking about their welfare might just enable them to cope with the procedure better.

Example from practice

McDougall *et al.* (2006) used a pre-test–post-test design to evaluate a community paediatric outreach team's effectiveness in relation to the care of children with acquired brain injury.

So, perhaps our design would be better if we had another group of participants who did not have (were not exposed to) the pre-testing. Then we could be sure that the pre-testing was not influencing the results from the post-testing.

So, here we go. In Figure 4.3, we have a group of participants who do not have the pre-testing.

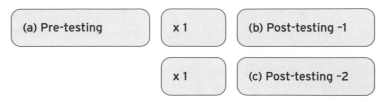

Figure 4.3 Research design using three groups of participants.

We probably now expect to see a difference between (a) and (b), but there should be no difference between (b) and (c). If there is a difference between (b) and (c), then we would suspect that the pre-testing has had an undesirable effect on our data. We should note, however, that this design is more expensive, because this design will need more participants and the researchers will have to do one more testing. We should also bear in mind that we may simply not have available sufficient participants to enable the use of this design.

However, we are not through yet because we can think of another problem with our design. You may be wondering where the control group is. You are right: there could indeed be a problem with our design.

But why would we need a control group? After all, we can tell what happens between pre-testing and post-testing; surely whatever difference exists must be due to the intervention. Perhaps so, and there may be times when a control group is not warranted. A control group is going to be expensive and we shouldn't use one if we can make a convincing argument that it isn't needed.

Anyway, let's look at what a design with a control group can look like. The design in Figure 4.4, sometimes known as the Solomon four-group design (see Chapman and Richman 1998), can tell us:

(a) what difference exists before and after the intervention (experimental group 1);

(b) whether pre-testing is influencing post-testing scores (experimental group 2);

(c) whether the difference found in (a) would have occurred even without the intervention (control group 1);

(d) whether the effect found at post-testing was simply due to the passage of time (control group 2).

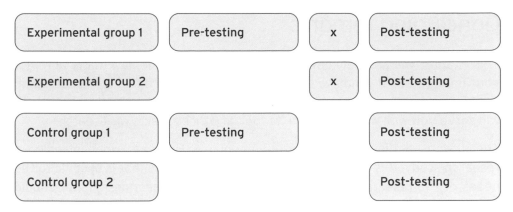

Figure 4.4 Research design using control groups.

If our researchers think that they do not need to test for an effect caused simply by the passage of time or of the effect of pre-testing, then a more simple design may be appropriate. Figure 4.5 shows a design sometimes referred to as the 'classic experimental design'.

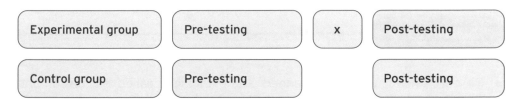

Figure 4.5 Classic experimental design.

There is no hard and fast rule about whether one needs to test for a particular effect, such as that of time (the passage of time) or of pre-testing. With each research project, it is necessary to make informed choices about what should be tested. Sometimes a more simple design is perfectly appropriate, and at other times a more complex and costly design is necessary. Perhaps the Solomon four-group design, with its ability to test for just about everything, is as close to perfection as we can usually get. However, it may test for things that are surplus to requirements and in so doing may make an unwarranted use of other people's time and money. Both time and money are often precious resources. A great deal of health research is funded by charitable income, and researchers have a duty to use the available funding wisely. For this reason, there is no perfect design, just a most appropriate one in a given situation.

Concluding remarks

This chapter will probably have presented you with some new material to get your head round. If you have found this chapter a little difficult to understand in places, read it again. A good understanding of the material in this chapter will serve you well when you come to look at other aspects of research.

The designs outlined here are in common use. However, when planning a research study, it is always necessary to create a design that is specific to the needs of the research study in question. There is no best design; nor should we choose a design just because it happens to be popular. When you design your house, you will not choose the most popular design, for you will want your house to be just as you want it to be. Your house may have to be energy-efficient or it may have to withstand storms or floods. Perhaps your house will need to keep out the heat of the day and be capable of collecting every last drop of rain. There is no best design, only a design that is fit for purpose and that does the job intended of it. So it is always necessary to think and use one's intelligence and imagination.

Summary

- Research needs to be well planned. The planning is called the 'design and methods' of a study.

- The plans need to be available after a study is complete, so that others can see how the study was undertaken and judge its quality.

- There are many designs used in clinical research, and these can look complex, largely because there are so many of them. This simply reflects that healthcare is a broad area of study. The many research designs in use reflect the fact that practitioners have become interested in a wide variety of phenomena and the many different ways in which patients' lives can be improved.

- There is no perfect design, only a design that is most fit for purpose in relation to the aims of any one particular research study.

- In determining the most appropriate design, the researcher needs to think carefully about what is to be achieved, what constraints exist and the degree to which any proposed design will produce a robust study.

Further reading

Examples of quantitative studies:

Meyers, T. A., D. J. Eichhorn, C. E. Guzzetta *et al.* (2004). 'Family presence during invasive procedures and resuscitation: the experience of family members, nurses, and physicians', reprinted with permission from the *American Journal of Nursing*, 2000; 100(2): 32-42'. *Topics in Emergency Medicine* **26**(1): 61-73.

Terry, L. M. and J. Carroll (2008). 'Dealing with death: first encounters for first-year nursing students'. *British Journal of Nursing (BJN)* **17**(12): 760-765.

Example of a phenomenological study:

Rosedale, M. (2009). 'Survivor loneliness of women following breast cancer'. *Oncology Nursing Forum* **36**(2): 175-183.

Example of grounded theory research:

Drury, V., K. Francis and Y. Chapman (2008). 'Mature learners becoming registered nurses: a grounded theory model'. *Australian Journal of Advanced Nursing* **26**(2): 39-45.

Example of ethnographical research:

Roberts, D. (2008). 'Learning in clinical practice: the importance of peers'. *Nursing Standard* **23**(12): 35-41.

Example of a descriptive study (this one is qualitative):

Mackintosh, C. (2007). 'Making patients better: a qualitative descriptive study of registered nurses' reasons for working in surgical areas'. *Journal of Clinical Nursing* **16**(6): 1134-1140.

Example of a deductive study:

Fincham, F. and J. Jaspars (1979). 'Attribution of responsibility to the self and other in children and adults'. *Journal of Personality and Social Psychology* **37**(9): 1589-1602.

Example of an inductive study:

Maputle, M. S. and A. Nolte (2008). 'Mothers' experiences of labour in a tertiary care hospital'. *Health SA Gesondheid* **13**(1): 55-62.

Example of experimental research:

Edwards, H., A. Walsh, M. Courtney *et al.* (2007). 'Improving paediatric nurses' knowledge and attitudes in childhood fever management'. *Journal of Advanced Nursing* **57**(3): 257-269.

Example of explorative research (this one is qualitative):

Jeong, S. Y. and D. Keatinge (2004). 'Innovative leadership and management in a nursing home'. *Journal of Nursing Management* **12**(6): 445-451.

Examples of randomised control studies:

Jubb, R. W., E. S. Tukmachi, P. W. Jones *et al.* (2008). 'A blinded randomised trial of acupuncture (manual and electroacupuncture) compared with a non-penetrating sham for the symptoms of osteoarthritis of the knee'. *Acupuncture in Medicine* **26**(2): 69-78.

Harkin, C. and R. Parker (2007). 'A prospective, randomised control trial of acupuncture for select common conditions within the emergency department'. *Journal of Chinese Medicine* **85**: 41-48.

Example of a survey:

McCabe, A. and H. Duncan (2008). 'National survey of observation and monitoring practices of children in hospital'. *Paediatric Nursing* **20**(6): 24-27.

References

Chapman, M. V. and J. M. Richman (1998). 'Practice highlights: promoting research and evaluation of practice in school-based programs: lessons learned'. *Social Work in Education* **20**(3): 203-208.

Fincham, F. and J. Jaspars (1979). 'Attribution of responsibility to the self and other in children and adults'. *Journal of Personality and Social Psychology* **37**(9): 1589-1602.

Glaser, B. G. and A. Strauss (1967). *The Discovery of Grounded Theory: Strategies for Qualitative Research*. Chicago: Aldine.

Maputle, M. S. and A. Nolte (2008). 'Mothers' experiences of labour in a tertiary care hospital'. *Health SA Gesondheid* **13**(1): 55-62.

McDougall, J., M. Servais, J. Sommerfreund *et al.* (2006). 'An evaluation of the paediatric acquired brain injury community outreach programme (PABICOP)'. *Brain Injury* **20**(11): 1189–1205.

Oshodi, T. O. (2007). 'The impact of preoperative education on postoperative pain: part 1'. *British Journal of Nursing (BJN)* **16**(12): 706–710.

Piaget, J. (1952). *The Origins of Intelligence*. New York: Harcourt Brace.

Piaget, J. and B. Inhelder (1972). *The Psychology of the Child*. New York: Basic Books.

Roberts, D. (2008). 'Learning in clinical practice: the importance of peers'. *Nursing Standard* **23**(12): 35–41.

Rosedale, M. (2009). 'Survivor loneliness of women following breast cancer'. *Oncology Nursing Forum* **36**(2): 175–183.

Stevenson, G. (2003). *Palaces for the People: Prefabs in Post-War Britain*. London: Batsford.

Chapter 5
The nature and collection of data

CHAPTER OBJECTIVES

The objectives for this chapter are to:

- Distinguish between nominal, ordinal, interval and ratio levels of measurement

- Illustrate how different modes of questioning can lead to different levels of data

- Demonstrate how the levels of measurement are related to the proper choice of statistical procedure

- Discuss the use of qualitative data

- Introduce the most commonly used methods of collecting quantitative and qualitative data.

Chapter outline

In this chapter we will look at data, what they are and how they are collected. 'Data' is a collective term for the stuff that is collected by research. In this chapter we will look at the forms in which data exist before they are made subject to statistical or qualitative analysis. The fact is, not all data are the same. Of course, there are data that exist as numbers and data that exist as written or spoken words. However, a quick look at the different forms of data will bear much fruit later on in terms of our understanding of analysis and in relation to our understanding of research in general.

Once we have spent a page or two looking at the different kinds of data, we will be able to relax a little and briefly consider the various ways in which data can be collected.

What are data?

Numerical data

Essentially, data are the stuff that is collected during a research project. The data will be made subject to analysis. Data can exist in the form of numbers (in quantitative research) or as words (in qualitative research).

New words

Raw data Data before they are analysed – the actual stuff collected by researchers.

Datum A single piece of data, like a single number. The word 'datum' isn't found much in the literature, but the plural form 'data' gives rise to some rather odd sounding sentences such as 'the data were analysed'.

So why are data important? Why not just look at results? We can just look at the results of a study, but understanding the kind of data used will help us to make sense of the results. There are different kinds of data, and the kind of data used in a research study will determine the kind of analysis that is used. Let's look at some of the things that you know.

Qualitative data usually exist in the form of words, sometimes written words, sometimes spoken words, but words in some form or another. We cannot easily use statistics with words. We cannot ask, for example, what is the average of 'happy' and 'sad', and we cannot easily add happy to sad. So, some forms of analysis fit with some forms of data and not with other forms of data.

There are some forms of analysis that do not work with some forms of numerical data. So, we can add up the number of males and we can add up the number of females. Let us say that there are 15 men and 15 women in our sample – so then the average sex is '15'? You already know that that doesn't make sense. So, there are some statistical procedures that cannot be used with some forms of data.

The sort of data we have fit with the analysis that is required. Understanding this can help us to make sense of the analysis. When a research project is planned, the researcher will identify the kind of data that the study will produce and will then identify the appropriate analysis. This is important because not every kind of data can be analysed as we might want – remember, however big our sample, even if we were able to sample every male and every female in the world, we will never be able to calculate an average sex because there will always be just so many males and so many females.

This is more serious than it sounds; look at the next example. Let us say that we want to measure the amount of pain experienced by patients after they have sustained a fractured femur. Foolishly, we ask 1000 patients: 'Do you have any pain?' We find that 999 patients say 'Yes' and one says 'No' (that patient had actually come into hospital for an eye test but had accidentally joined the queue of patients with a fractured femur because he couldn't read the signs well enough).

So, how much pain did the patients have? Well, we don't know; we asked them only whether they had pain. These kind of 'yes/no' data do not give us very much information, even though we have a sample of 1000 people. In circumstances like this, people say that the data are not 'rich' or not 'deep'.

It is worth bearing in mind that if we collect 'shallow' data, we may not be able to do much with them. You may think that no one would choose to collect such shallow data, but you would be wrong to make such an assumption. When you read the research literature, you should question whether the data collected really were the best that could have been collected. Practitioners collect data all the time as they assess patients and clients and make decisions about them. Imagine that you can see a patient being admitted to an orthopaedic ward. Look at the nurse who kindly and sympathetically approaches the new patient and asks 'Have you any pain?' Oops!

So how should we ask patients about their pain? You may have used a pain scale of some sort or another. Figure 5.1 shows a pain scale that is often used with children.

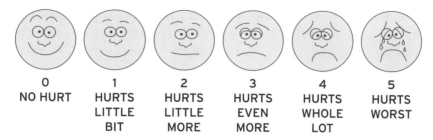

Figure 5.1 Wong-Baker FACES pain rating scale.
Source: Hockenberry MJ, Wilson D, Winkelstein ML: *Wong's Essentials of Pediatric Nursing*, 7th edn. St Louis, 2005, p. 1259. Used with permission. Copyright, Mosby.

So now we have a scale; in this case, the scale is quite short (0-5) but it still allows us to:

- determine a mean score for pain;[1]

- develop at least some idea of whether there is a little pain or a lot of pain;

- determine differences between groups of people in relation to pain; for example, we can determine whether pain worsens or improves with a nursing procedure.

Some scales are longer than 1-5. These longer scales can give us richer information. Imagine, for example, that your sphygmomanometer[2] gives readings only between 1 and 5. You will agree that that would not be a good thing. Sometimes a patient's systolic blood pressure (BP) may be as low as 40 mmHg (this patient is clearly not very well) or as high as 250 mmHg (this patient is not very well either). That's quite a big scale. In fact, the scale on which we measure BP doesn't really have any ends to it; it can even be negative – like the pressure in the veins in your legs if you were to hang yourself upside down like a bat. Perhaps we could simplify the scale, but would you want to do that? It can be quite useful to know that the patient's BP has gone up from 40 mmHg to 45 mmHg – at least the patient is improving. Apparently minor moves up and down a scale can be important. So, sometimes long scales are useful as they offer seriously rich data.

We have seen that some forms of data give us more information than do other forms of data. Not all data are the same. We have used numerical examples here, but exactly the same is true of qualitative data. Here, we can ask someone

---

[1] The mean should be used with care when the scale is not continuous. The mean in this case could be returned as 5.5 (for example) or a number half way between 5 and 6. Yet, it is not possible for a patient to choose such a number.

[2] A sphygmomanometer is a blood pressure recording machine.

whether they have pain, and we record the verbal response, 'yes' or 'no'; or perhaps the patient will say 'I have a little niggle' or 'My big toe really hurts when I walk on it.' These responses are qualitative data. Try adding up three little niggles and a big toe – it just doesn't work – but the responses are data all the same; they have meaning to us, meaning that is shared between the patient and ourselves. These data exist as a common understanding. However, the data are pretty shallow and most qualitative researchers would turn up their nose at such a form of enquiry (Baker 2006). The qualitative researcher is more likely to ask 'Tell me about your pain' or perhaps 'How do you feel when you have pain?' (Whiting 2008). Such questions are likely to yield data that are rich (or deep).

Types of quantitative data

There are three main types of numerical data:

- *Categories* – called 'nominal' data
- *Small scales* – called 'ordinal' data
- *Long scales* – called 'interval' or 'ratio' data.

These four terms, nominal, ordinal, interval and ratio, are sometimes referred to as 'levels of measurement' (Vojir *et al.* 2006). They are really levels of data. Interval and ratio are deeper levels (rich in information), and nominal is a relatively shallow level, offering less depth of data. Here are some examples.

Nominal level of measurement – categories

- Yes/no questions
- Discrete categories, such as: Are you male or female? Are you tall, middle-sized or short?

Sometimes, a range of categories can look like a small scale:

Normally, do you drink:

(a) No alcohol?

(b) Up to 2 units of alcohol per day?

(c) More than 2 units of alcohol per day?

In practice, however, a scale with fewer than 5 points on it is usually regarded as categorical (as discrete categories and not as a scale). It would be possible to calculate a mean from the data produced by the alcohol question above, but the result would not be quite as meaningful as we might like. If we assigned numbers 1, 2 and 3 to the responses, we might find that our 'average' score was (for example) 1.5 - that is, somewhere between 'no alcohol' and 'up to two units per day'. However, we would need to bear in mind that no one would have given such an answer. In this example, the 'average' score does not really make sense.

Nominal level data have a range of statistical procedures available to them, which tend not to be used on ordinal, interval or ratio data. An example of such a statistical procedure is the Pearson chi square, which can be used to test for differences between, for example, two groups of categorical data, in the form:

Particular preference for wearing a uniform	Yes	No
Females	12	4
Males	5	12

In this completely fictitious example, 17 males and 16 females were asked whether they wanted to wear a uniform or to wear their own clothes at work. We can see here that there is a relationship between the responses given by males and females. Males in this fictitious example were more likely to respond 'no' and females were more likely to respond 'yes'. The data here are categorical - that is, they exist in categories and are therefore at the nominal level of measurement. Perhaps the data here are not very rich or deep; we don't, for example, know why our fictitious males wanted to wear their own clothes at work or the strength of feeling they had on the matter. However, these data are useful here. Sometimes categorical data are all that we have available to use - males are males and females are females and that is that. Sometimes, categories do tell us all we need to know about something. Statistical procedures such as the Pearson chi square are available for use on categorical data. In fact, if we ran a Pearson chi square on the data here, we would get the result 5.155, with $P = 0.0232$.[3] Don't worry about the numbers just yet; they mean, however, that the difference we see here between the responses

---

[3] Chi square with Yates correction, two-tailed.

of males and females is not likely to be caused simply by chance – that is, it is not a chance finding. Some people would describe this result as 'significant'.

So, Pearson chi square can work for nominal level (categorical) data. Not all statistical procedures work here though. Consider one of the most simple statistical procedures – the mean, or average. Try to apply the average to the data in the preference for wearing a uniform box above; you will probably not make much useful progress.

Ordinal level of measurement – ranking and short scales

The ordinal level of measurement is so named because it is meant to be used with a list of possible responses that are placed in order – that is, they are ranked. Here is a list of things that the research participant could be asked to order.

What causes you most pain? Please place in order, with [1] at the top of the list causing most pain:

- Getting up in the morning

- Walking

- Running

- Having to bend down

- Having to move after a period of sitting or resting.

Such ordinal lists can give us some quite useful information (data). In practice, however, the lists are usually quite short. Imagine having to place in order a list with 100 items on it. On the other hand, these ordinal lists are longer than those we looked at in the nominal level of measurement. In a way, these lists form a short scale. This is important because, over the years, a range of statistical procedures has been developed for ordinal lists that work just as well for any short scale.

Short scales are often used in research, largely because research participants find them easier to work with than they do longer scales. Perhaps the most commonly used short scale is a Likert scale.[4] A Likert scale presents the research participant with a statement and then asks the participant to choose a response from a list. Here is an example.

[4] First proposed by Rensis Likert (1903–1981).

I think that NHS dentists should be available to everyone:

1. Strongly disagree

2. Disagree

3. Neither agree nor disagree

4. Agree

5. Strongly agree.

The data resulting from this short scale are probably best analysed using a range of statistical procedures designed for the ordinal level of measurement. This is the case, even though such short scales do not require ranking (placing in order).

Ordinal-level data have a range of statistical procedures that have been designed just for them. An example is the Mann–Whitney U statistical procedure, which is used when we want to test differences between two groups of data, each produced using a short scale (ordinal level data) (Crichton 2000).

Interval level of measurement – long scales

Your essays are probably marked on a scale from 0 to 100. This is quite a long scale. In fact, it is so long that it is effectively continuous. It is true that you (probably) cannot be awarded a score of 55.789%, but there are so many points in the scale 0–100 that points between any two numbers would be meaningless to most of us.

These longer scales provide richer data. If your academic work was marked on a scale of 1–5, you might begin to be dissatisfied with the meaningfulness of the mark. You might, for example, want your university to distinguish between those people who got a 'lower three' and those who 'nearly got a four'. There is no correct length of scale for every purpose. We have to determine for ourselves what length of scale produces data that are meaningful to us and what length gives us the richness of data that we think is appropriate.

Degree classifications are usually of the form:

● First class

● Upper second class

- Lower second class

- Third class

- Pass.

This seems to work well for most people. However, the poor student who gets 1 mark under a first-class degree (usually 70% overall) might well feel unhappy that the overall percentage mark is not printed on their degree certificate.

There is no perfect length for a scale. It is up to us to determine what length of scale is fit for purpose. However, it is always the case that longer scales give us more information. Interval-level data have a rather larger range of statistical procedures available to them than is the case for either nominal (categories) or ordinal (short-scale) data. This reflects the increased richness of interval-level data. We would probably not use the Mann–Whitney U procedure for two groups of data as we did for ordinal (short-scale) data; rather, we might use a procedure called the Student's *t*-test. Don't worry about all these statistical procedures just yet, but do bear in mind that different kinds of data often require different statistical procedures. It is not important to be able to remember which statistical procedure fits with which kind of data, but it is useful to understand that not all data are the same and that at some point we will need to be sure that the most appropriate statistical test is used.

Ratio level of measurements – long scales without any ends

We have already come across ratio data. These are simply data that have no top and no bottom. We have noted that blood pressure can be below zero sometimes and can be as high as you like. You can't get more than 100% for your examinations because those data are interval and have a known bottom (0%) and a known top (100%). However, data in the form of blood pressure, body temperature, bacterial counts and blood alcohol have no limits. In practice, a bacterial count of −1 is a little difficult to construe, but at the top end it can be just about anything. Blood pressure over 500 mmHg is probably not compatible with life. However, there is a real difference between these scales and the one used for your examinations. Ratio-level data do exist. However, effectively, and in practice, interval- and ratio-level data are treated exactly the same. If we know interval-level data, then we know ratio data, and the statistical procedures used for one can be used with the other.

Numbers – summary

Just a little effort with the question of the different types of numerical data (numbers) will help a lot with our grasp of research in general. Numbers can be confusing. However, let us review what we have learned here.

There are essentially four levels of data:

- *Nominal*: categories, such as yes/no

- *Ordinal*: ranked data or short scales, such as a Likert scale

- *Interval*: longer scales, where the middle ground between, say 57% and 58%, is effectively meaningless

- *Ratio*: just like interval data but without a known top and bottom to the scale.

These levels are important because they relate to:

- the richness of the data;

- the choice of statistical tools available to us.

Researchers are sometimes limited to a particular level of measurement (such as ordinal) where the data only ever exist at that level. However, sometimes researchers can select data collection tools that will yield data at a particular level of measurement. In this way, the researcher can require the participant to respond with 'yes' or 'no' or can use questioning with a short or a long scale. In this case, the choice is important because it relates directly to the range of statistical procedures available to the analysis and the 'amount' of information that the data are able to yield.

Types of qualitative data

Qualitative data take the form of words or meanings. The data can be taken from written communications or verbal dialogue but can also take the form of still or moving images, ideas, drawings and anything that is capable of being summarised and interpreted. Some people will question the scientific nature of qualitative data, but it is suggested here that qualitative data can be and are handled scientifically. In addition, we have noted already that qualitative data are often used to explore situations that could not be explored quantitatively.

However, numbers can be used to explore meanings. In fact, we have already come across an example of this.

I think that NHS dentists should be available to everyone:

1. Strongly disagree

2. Disagree

3. Neither agree nor disagree

4. Agree

5. Strongly agree

This is a Likert scale. It is being used here to obtain data on people's views on the provision of NHS dentistry. In this example, a number is being assigned to a notion, idea or viewpoint. This can work well when we know what the notions, ideas or viewpoints are. It probably works well here. We know what range of views exist about the provision of NHS dentists, or we can at least take an educated guess at what views exist. In essence, the research participants, the data collector and the data analyst are all likely to be speaking the same language; they understand each other. So, a whole range of feelings, emotions, experiences and all things human can be and often are explored quantitatively – using numbers.

Qualitative research comes into its own when, basically, we don't know what questions to ask and where a shared and meaningful communication with the research participant is not at all straightforward. Healthcare practitioners are often interested in the things that make their patients and clients psychologically uncomfortable. These things often exist as experiences that trouble the patient or client in some way. Consider, for example, the experience of having a child in the intensive care unit (ICU) or the experience of someone who is in grief or distress.

If we could know how parents felt about having a child in the ICU, then we might be better able to help them. The trouble is, most of us don't know what it is like. We can guess, but most of us would be conscious that we might guess incorrectly. We are often quick to suggest that we don't know how someone else feels. It can be difficult to 'get inside someone's head' and see things the way they see them. Qualitative research is good at exploring feelings, notions, experiences, etc., which we don't know very much about.

Not only do we not know what the individual is feeling but also we know so little about it that we don't even know what questions to ask. Structured questions seem particularly inappropriate. Consider the following questions asked by our fictitious nurse admitting a child to ICU. The questions are directed to the child's mother:

- How old is Benjamin?

- Is he on any special diet?

- Does he have any special words (e.g. for 'toilet') of which we should be aware?

And then:

- Are you not anxious ☐, a little anxious ☐ or very anxious ☐?

- Do you think that Benjamin will die? Yes ☐, No ☐

Of course, this is not appropriate: the nurse would not ask these questions and neither would the researcher. There are two reasons for this.

- We do not know what the child's mother is experiencing, so we don't know what to ask her about.

- Even if we think we know what sort of things she is experiencing, we are uncomfortable about putting these into preconceived or artificial categories. In this example, we do not know whether Benjamin's mother is thinking about his possible death; she may not have construed events in this way. There may be other thoughts that are important to Benjamin's mother and that it would be useful to know about. In asking Benjamin's mother about death, the nurse is putting thoughts inside the mother's head. Here, the nurse is impacting on the mother's construction of reality. In clinical practice, this is not good; in research, it is very damaging. We want to know what the mother is thinking about, not what she is thinking about after ideas have been suggested to her by a third party.

In asking these questions, we run the risk of insulting the participant or patient, in the way that our question can suggest an answer. One does not ask 'Do you think that Benjamin will die?' without suggesting to the mother that this is something she *ought* to be thinking of. Clearly, the researcher and the nurse should want to find out what is going on in the participant's head, not what the researcher can put there.

In practice, the nurse would be sensitive about his or her own lack of knowledge of what is going on in the mother's mind. Being so sensitive, she might ask:

- Tell me how you feel.

- Is there anything that you would like to say to me just now?

Questions such as these might enable the child's mother to communicate her feelings freely and without being constrained by artificially contrived questions. The nurse and the child's mother can potentially come to a shared understanding of what is being experienced. This is exactly the way it is with research.

So, qualitative research does have a useful purpose (Wiart and Burwash 2007). It is widely employed in healthcare, perhaps because practitioners often want to reach a better understanding of their patients' and clients' experiences. It follows that the data in qualitative research are usually focused on human experience. These data usually take the form of words, either spoken or written, but they can take any form from which interpretations can be discerned. For example, when Benjamin begins to get better, the nurse might give him paper and pencils and Benjamin might explore his own feelings through drawings (Matsumori 2005; Jolley 2010). Benjamin might find this easier than speaking because he still has an endotracheal tube in his airway or perhaps because, being only 4 years old, he's not so good at expressing the nuances of his experience in words. Once again, the researcher may well use the same approach – children's drawings have been used to help explore their experiences of violence, of war and of serious illness (Hatlevig 2006; Jolley 2010).

Ways of collecting data

When one begins to look at published research, it soon becomes apparent that data are collected using a variety of means. However, understanding this is easy because you are already aware of these different means.

Here are some of the most popular ways of collecting data. (note that, in each case, the method of collecting the data influences the kind of data that are obtained):

- Questionnaire
- Interview
- Participant and non-participant observation
- Existing data and meta-analyses
- Historical data and records
- Audio, film and photographic records.

It is important to understand that, although there are advantages and disadvantages associated with each type of data collection, there is no right or wrong way to collect data. As with every other aspect of research, there is no right or wrong way to do this, only the most appropriate way, considering what it is that the research project in question aims to achieve. It is worth emphasising this point because people new to research are sometimes too ready to criticise a research project on the basis that the use of interviews, for example, carries some disadvantages. Interviews *do* have disadvantages, but they may still be the best and perhaps the only way of collecting data in respect of what a particular research project is trying to achieve.

Let's look at each data collection method in a little more detail.

The questionnaire

You will probably be familiar with questionnaires. Most of us occasionally receive them in the post or online, get stopped in the street to answer questions or have come across questionnaires at some other point. Almost by definition, a questionnaire is a written thing containing one or more kinds of question. The questionnaire may be presented on paper or, increasingly, may be available electronically. The questionnaire is simply a means of communication, often used because data can be collected efficiently and inexpensively. It is not difficult to post out thousands of questionnaires to people, who will then (we assume) sit patiently, complete the form and obediently post it back to us. In the same way, web-based questionnaires can easily reach many thousands of people. In this case, the data can be collected electronically and even analysed automatically. So, let's be clear about this: questionnaires can be very useful. Indeed, it is for this reason that they are so much in use.

Questionnaires can contain questions designed to yield nominal (categories), ordinal (short-scale) or interval (long-scale) data (Rattray and Jones 2007). Here are three questions that deal with each in turn:

(Q1) Are you male ☐ or female ☐ ?

(Q2) Place in order of preference the following activities:

Watching the TV ☐

Walking ☐

Playing your favourite sport ☐

Going to the gym ☐

Sunbathing ☐

(Q3) What is your yearly income (state amount) [£_____] ?

So, questionnaires are pretty good at eliciting data at all the levels of measurement discussed earlier in this chapter. However, questionnaires can also be used to obtain qualitative data, as in:

(Q4) What do you think would most encourage you to get more exercise?

Now, some people would regard this as merely an open-ended question. The term 'qualitative research' is probably best left to situations where meanings can be shared between at least two people. The question here is open-ended: the participant can answer as he or she pleases but the question does still have structure (the question could have said 'Tell me what you think about exercise') and, importantly, there can be no dialogue between the researcher and the participant. In qualitative research, it is important to achieve a shared understanding of what is being communicated. A questionnaire can never fully facilitate this because it is not possible for the researcher to probe the participant. Let us say that a participant has responded to question 4 as follows:

(Q4) What do you think would most encourage you to get more exercise?

I hated sports and physical education at school and that has put me off doing any form of exercise now.

Now, it might be good to explore this with the participant, but a questionnaire does not make such an exploration easy. Arguably, questionnaires are best used to collect data from closed or structured questions or when achieving a common understanding with the participant is relatively unproblematic.

You may have had experience of a questionnaire that is hard to understand. If you have had to apply for a UK passport recently, you may be familiar with the problem. It is important that the questions in a questionnaire are meaningful, both to the participant and to the researcher. Consider this question, included in a fictitious questionnaire to student nurses:

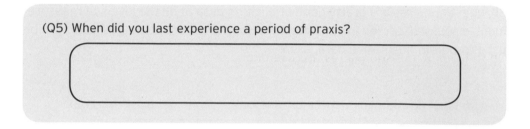

(Q5) When did you last experience a period of praxis?

Well, what do you think: is this a question about the menstrual period? Dysmenorrhoea, perhaps. Not really: 'praxis' means the practical side of professional activity, and so the question means 'When did you last have a clinical placement?' It is easy for words to be misunderstood and this can cause real problems in research. Imagine this: the poor researcher thinks the study will reveal all sorts of juicy information about clinical placements, but all the study reveals is how much dysmenorrhoea there is about.

The main disadvantage of questionnaires is that there is often no facility to interact with the participant. However, questionnaires can be used during face-to-face meetings. Sometimes these exist simply to ensure that all sections of the questionnaire are completed and that the participant understands the questions being asked. When someone stops you in the street and asks you for a few minutes of your time to fill in a questionnaire, the chances are that the researcher will complete the questionnaire. There may be only a limited dialogue between the researcher and the participant, but it is sufficient to ensure that the participant understands the questions.

There is another problem that is sometimes associated with the use of questionnaires; we cannot always tell whether the participants have been truthful. There are all manner of reasons that people don't always want to tell the truth. An individual might not be too truthful about how much exercise they get each day, how much alcohol they drink or when they first had sex. After all, these questions can be perceived as personal. In practice, participants can leave questions unanswered if they don't want to answer them, but all too often they may give us a response that is not true. Researchers don't usually talk about 'truth'; rather, they use the word 'validity'. There are ways in which one can test the validity of questionnaire data. One might ask the same question twice but re-worded slightly, or one might repeat a question on another occasion. A lot is written about validity. The fact remains, though: it is difficult to discern whether a participant lies reliably (consistently). This may be a problem with any kind of data collection, but it is perhaps more of a problem where the researcher and the participant are not working together, as in the case of a postal questionnaire.

On the whole, questionnaires are useful and there are many occasions when they work well. However, as with any kind of data collection, one always needs to question whether there might be a better way of collecting the data. Whether there is or not will usually depend on what the research project in question is trying to achieve.

The interview

This one-to-one communication gets round a lot of the problems associated with the questionnaire. A one-to-one dialogue can ensure that what is communicated is understood by both parties – that is, that there is a common understanding. The interview also enables a less structured, more flexible and more in-depth gathering of data. The interview makes it possible to probe the participant (but not physically!). In the best interviews, the participant and the researcher have a common goal of reaching a shared understanding of the participant's views or experiences.

The main disadvantage of interviews is that they are time-consuming and resource-intensive. However, the interview should not be dismissed just because it is resource-intensive. If the interview is the most effective way of collecting data, then interviews should be used. The real question is whether the data could be collected more easily or less expensively in some other way. As always, whether it can or not will depend on what the research study is aiming to achieve.

The interview is probably best used where a shared understanding has to be worked at and where a shared understanding does not come naturally or easily (DiCicco-Bloom and Crabtree 2006). It is not surprising, then, that the interview is often used in qualitative studies. Having said that, interviews are often appropriate in quantitative studies too. Consider the admission interview or pre-admission interview often undertaken by nurses. Here, the nurse asks the patient questions about a range of things, from current health status to who will look after the dog when the patient comes into hospital. Now, it would be possible to send the patient a pre-admission questionnaire, but there are advantages in seeing the patient, not least because it allows any concerns to be probed.

Let's emphasise this point one more time – there is no perfect method of collecting data, only the most effective method in relation to what the study in question aims to achieve.

Participant and non-participant observation

So far, we have looked at methods of data collection that rely on participants' accounts of something that has taken place or on their views or experiences of something. Sometimes, however, the researcher will want to make a direct observation of something that is taking place. So, for example, it is possible to watch healthcare staff washing their hands between procedures to take an objective measurement of the standard of hand-washing.

'Participant observation' is a term used to describe a situation where the re-searcher is involved in the situation being measured; in this case, the researcher would be a nurse who would be washing his or her hands, along with the other staff. The nurse researcher might do this 'covertly' (secretly), although these days covert data collection raises a number of ethical concerns and does not tend to be practised. Usually, then, the staff being watched know that they are being watched and have agreed to this. Non-participant observation takes place when the researcher is not involved directly in the practice being measured.

Both participant and non-participant observation can raise concerns about something called the Hawthorne effect[5] (or sometimes performance bias). The Hawthorne effect is where the behaviour of those being watched changes because they know they are being watched. In the case of our nurses, for example, we may find that they take extra care to wash their hands according to the hospital procedure. There are a number of ways to counter the Hawthorne effect, the most usual being for the researcher to be present for some time before data are actually collected. In this way, the behaviour of the individuals concerned eventually returns to normal as they become used to (habituated to) the presence of the researcher(s). Cutler and Davis (2005) used this technique when measuring the quality of oral hygiene performed in intensive care.

The Hawthorne effect is an example (in a sense) of participants being less than honest with the researcher. We have come across this problem before when we looked at the use of questionnaires, but we have perhaps seen here that the problem of honesty pervades most kinds of data collection. In a sense, we do not entirely escape the problem, even where we may, for example, want to count bacteria on nurses' hands as a measure of their hand-washing skills. The bacteria are not going to clump together in one heap just because they know they are being watched, but we do have to consider how reliable has been our sampling of the bacteria. So, validity (the extent to which the data are the data

[5] The Hawthorne effect is so named because it was first identified in studies that took place at the Hawthorne Works, a factory outside Chicago. The effect was first described by Henry Landsberger.

we think they are) and reliability (the degree to which the results would be the same if we did the research again) are related concepts at the heart of any research study. Every research study needs to address the degree to which the study can demonstrate validity and reliability. There are ways of measuring validity and reliability (Salmond 2008), but these are far from perfect and each research study should be critiqued in relation to what risks exist that the data may not be what we think they are.

Participant and non-participant observation are resource-intensive means of collecting data. Typically, the process will involve months of work with the participants even before the data collection begins (see Cutler and Davis 2005). There are ethical considerations in watching people and recording what they do, and today's media-sensitive NHS does not always welcome researchers who wish to carry out these modes of data collection.

Participant and non-participant observation remain useful techniques in healthcare research and where we want to study the behaviour or performance of nurses or patients. Again, let's make the point that it is not a case of which data collection type is 'best' but rather which mode of data collection is most appropriate, considering what the research project in question aims to achieve.

Existing data and meta-analyses

It has always been possible to take existing data and subject those data to analysis. Sometimes the data from existing studies are re-analysed, either to check on the original analysis or to run a different analysis. More usually, data that have not already been analysed will be used. An example of this is the analysis of census data, which takes place in various studies (Doran *et al.* 2003). Another example is the use of existing hospital records (Ansell *et al.* 2007). In both of these examples, the researchers in question have not had to collect their data as such. This means that there are fewer ethical issues with which the researchers have had to deal, though there may still be concerns over the researchers having access to the data, confidentiality and whether the data are likely to be held securely and eventually published.

Using existing data is not only a convenient route to data collection; it is also the most appropriate route in situations where the data already exist. It would be a waste of time collecting new data when existing data are available.

An important and relatively new way of using existing data is in the meta-analysis associated with systematic reviews. Systematic reviews have been mentioned in Chapter 4 and are a review of existing research on a particular topic, together with an analysis of the pooled data from (often) several studies. We noted in Chapter 4 that a convenient source of systematic reviews is the Cochrane Library.

> ## Example from the literature and research
>
> An example of a systematic review is that by Stevens *et al.* (2004). This study examined the evidence that the administration of sucrose to neonates could act as a safe analgesia. The systematic review examined the range of existing studies that met set criteria for methodological quality, pooled the data from these studies and subjected the new data set to analysis.

Historical data

Any profession, including medicine or nursing, has history. In part, it is the historical depth of the discipline that gives it its professional feel. Understanding the history of each profession makes it possible for us to put the present in perspective. Our understanding of history also helps to prevent us from making the same old mistakes again and makes it possible for us to learn from what has gone before (Jolley 2006). Apart from all of this, the history of healthcare can be a fascinating area to study.

Historical studies can involve searching through archives (Hilton 2005) or they can involve speaking with older people to find out what kind of things happened in the past.

> ## Example from the literature and research
>
> Jolley (2007) interviewed older people who either worked as children's nurses or who were child patients between 1920 and 1970 to examine their different perspectives of hospital care in that period.

Concluding remarks

If we can understand the different forms that data can take, then we will find that such knowledge illuminates our study of the other aspects of research. If you have been unsure of this chapter, read it again. What has been discussed here is not difficult to understand, but it is important that you understand it.

So we now know that there are different forms of data (levels of measurement). Numerical data exist as nominal (categories), ordinal (ranking or small scales), interval (long scales) and ratio (long scales without ends). As we move from nominal through to ratio, the data become deeper or richer – that is, they contain more information. Researchers need to acquire data that are at least rich enough to be fit for purpose. We have also noted that different levels of measurement (nominal, ordinal, etc.) fit with different statistical procedures. All this needs to be taken into account when research is planned.

We have looked briefly at qualitative data and seen how they can be used to help us measure such things as experiences, feelings and points of view.

From time to time, we have used examples of the way in which practitioners ask questions. We can use such examples to define research because there really isn't any difference between practice and research. In clinical practice, the practitioner is always asking questions and working to solve problems. So it is with research: practice and research are simply two sides of one approach to care. Data may not seem to be much fun, but when they are used within research they come alive.

Summary

- Qualitative data usually exist in the form of words rather than numbers. They are often derived from the researcher's attempts to explore feelings and emotions.

- Not all quantitative data are the same. The levels of measurement – that is, nominal (categories), ordinal (short-scale) and interval/ratio (longer-scale) – are important to understand because they determine both the depth of the data (potentially, how much the data tell us) and what statistical procedures can be used on the data.

- There isn't a best sort of data. Sometimes qualitative data better suit the purpose of the research than do quantitative data. Whatever form the data take, they should fit the overall aim of the research study.

- The kind of data generated by a study must be linked both to the planned analysis and to the specific objectives of the research. It follows that thought must be given to the sort of data that the study will generate at a time when the design and methods of the study are being decided.

Further reading

An introduction to qualitative research:

Smythe, L. and L. S. Giddings (2007). 'From experience to definition: addressing the question "What is qualitative research?"'. *Nursing Praxis in New
Zealand* **23**(1): 37-57.

The argument for the full legitimacy of qualitative research:

Wiart, L. and S. Burwash (2007). 'Qualitative research is evidence, too'.
Australian Journal of Physiotherapy **53**(4): 215-216.

A guide to critiquing quantitative research:

Coughlan, M., P. Cronin and F. Ryan (2007). 'Step-by-step guide to critiquing
research: part 1 - quantitative research'. *British Journal of Nursing (BJN)*
16(11): 658-663.

A guide to critiquing qualitative research:

Ryan, F., M. Coughlan and P. Cronin (2007). 'Step-by-step guide to critiquing
research: part 2 - qualitative research'. *British Journal of Nursing (BJN)*
16(12): 738-744.

An interesting account of a nurse's early experience of being involved in qualitative research:

Katsuno, T. (2006). 'Being a qualitative researcher in nursing'. *Japan Journal
of Nursing Science* **3**(1): 5-7.

A research paper showing the use of the chi square and the Mann-Whitney
statistical procedures to test the effectiveness of acupuncture:

Jubb, R. W., E. S. Tukmachi, P. W. Jones *et al.* (2008). 'A blinded randomised
trial of acupuncture (manual and electroacupuncture) compared with a
non-penetrating sham for the symptoms of osteoarthritis of the knee'.
Acupuncture in Medicine **26**(2): 69-78.

An introductory paper about questionnaire design:

Meadows, K. A. (2003). 'So you want to do research? 5: questionnaire design'.
British Journal of Community Nursing **8**(12): 562-570.

A more advanced paper about questionnaire design:

Rattray, J. and M. C. Jones (2007). 'Essential elements of questionnaire design and development'. *Journal of Clinical Nursing* **16**(2): 234-243.

A paper about research interviews:

DiCicco-Bloom, B. and B. F. Crabtree (2006). 'The qualitative research interview'. *Medical Education* **40**(4): 314-321.

An example of a systematic review and the use of existing data in new research:

Stevens, B., J. Yamada and A. Ohlsson (2004). 'Sucrose for analgesia in newborn infants undergoing painful procedures'. *Cochrane Database of Systematic Reviews* 2004 (3): CD001069.

A paper on historical research methodologies:

Sweeney, J. F. (2005). 'Historical research: examining documentary sources'. *Nurse Researcher* **12**(3): 61-73.

References

Ansell, P., D. Howell, A. Garry *et al.* (2007). 'What determines referral of UK patients with haematological malignancies to palliative care services? An exploratory study using hospital records'. *Palliative Medicine* **21**(6): 487–492.

Baker, L. (2006). 'Ten common pitfalls to avoid when conducting qualitative research'. *British Journal of Midwifery* **14**(9): 530-531.

Crichton, N. (2000). 'Information point: Mann–Whitney test'. *Journal of Clinical Nursing* **9**(4): 583.

Cutler, C. J. and N. Davis (2005). 'Improving oral care in patients receiving mechanical ventilation'. *American Journal of Critical Care* **14**(5): 389-394.

DiCicco-Bloom, B. and B. F. Crabtree (2006). 'The qualitative research interview'. *Medical Education* **40**(4): 314-321.

Doran, T., F. Drever and M. Whitehead (2003). 'Health of young and elderly informal carers: analysis of UK census data'. *British Medical Journal* **327**(7428): 1388.

Hatlevig, J. (2006). 'Children's life transition following sexual abuse'. *Journal of Forensic Nursing* **2**(4): 165-174.

Hilton, C. (2005). 'The clinical psychiatry of late life in Britain from 1950 to 1970: an overview'. *International Journal of Geriatric Psychiatry* **20**(5): 423-428.

Jolley, J. (2006). 'The progress of care'. *Paediatric Nursing* **18**(8): 12.

Jolley, J. (2007). Separation and psychological trauma: a paradox examined'. *Paediatric Nursing* **19**(3): 22-25.

Jolley, R. (2010). *Children and Pictures: Drawing and Understanding*. Chichester: John Wiley & Sons.

Matsumori, N. (2005). 'Ask the expert: use of the drawing technique in nursing assessment'. *Journal for Specialists in Pediatric Nursing* **10**(4): 191-195.

Rattray, J. and M. C. Jones (2007). 'Essential elements of questionnaire design and development'. *Journal of Clinical Nursing* **16**(2): 234-243.

Salmond, S. S. (2008). 'Taking the mystery out of research: evaluating the reliability and validity of measurement instruments'. *Orthopaedic Nursing* **27**(1): 28-30.

Stevens, B., J. Yamada and A. Ohlsson (2004). 'Sucrose for analgesia in newborn infants undergoing painful procedures'. *Cochrane Database of Systematic Reviews* 2004 (3): CD001069.

Vojir, C. P., K. R. Jones, R. Fink and E. Hutt (2006). 'Scientific inquiry'. *Journal for Specialists in Pediatric Nursing* **11**(4): 257-259.

Whiting, L. S. (2008). 'Semi-structured interviews: guidance for novice researchers'. *Nursing Standard* **22**(23): 35-40.

Wiart, L. and S. Burwash (2007). 'Qualitative research is evidence, too'. *Australian Journal of Physiotherapy* **53**(4): 215-216.

Chapter 6
Quantitative analysis

CHAPTER OBJECTIVES

The objectives for this chapter are to:

- Demonstrate that little or no knowledge of mathematics is required

- Provide the reader with the opportunity to practise doing some data analysis

- Illustrate the ways in which qualitative analysis is objective and rational

- Introduce the analyses used in Cochrane systematic reviews.

Chapter outline

This chapter will look at the use of analytical tools to describe data and to demonstrate the effect that one variable may have on another. The notion of probability will be introduced using examples with which you will probably be familiar. In fact, you will find that you are already fully conversant with the notion and use of probability. Using practical examples, this chapter will demonstrate the use of probability within research. The notion of proof will be examined, and it will be suggested that research seldom proves anything but merely determines the degree to which the results can be trusted.

One of the most scary aspects of research is the statistical analysis that is so often equated with research. This chapter will show that, in fact, very few mathematical skills need to be acquired to perform statistical tests.

Analysing numerical data

Let's make it clear straight away that you do not need to know how to calculate a statistical analysis. In the same way, you do not need to know how a cardiac monitor produces its display or even how your MP3 player works. It works and that's all you need to know. There are people who spend their lives studying the electronics inside the MP3 player and the maths inside statistical procedures. Our happy lot is to use the tools that these people devise for us. So, you can put your paper and pencil away now. Researchers do not calculate statistical analysis with a pencil and paper; they use a computer and they use programs on the computer that have been designed to produce statistical output. These programs are like word processors for numbers.

Statistical analysis is analysis; it is used to help us to clarify the nature of the data and to find things that might be hidden in the data, to find new information that is not clear without the analysis. For this to be successful, we need to know what it is that we want to find out. This is very similar to the problem-solving used in the nursing process. Before we work out what intervention is needed, we have to identify the problem. In analysis of numerical data, we need to be just as focused and just as clear about what it is we are looking for. It is not possible to run a series of randomly selected statistical analyses and then step back and see what happens.

There are two kinds of statistical procedure: descriptive and inferential. Descriptive statistics serve only to summarise data. The mean or average is a descriptive statistic, as is sum or total. To understand how old we are, we add up the years – so I am 55. This is my total, the sum of my years. One simple but rather large number summarises all of my numbers.

Inferential statistics are designed to determine the degree to which we can be sure about the correlation or difference between sets of data. In practice, we want to know whether any difference that exists is caused simply by chance or whether it is because of the effect of the variable that we think may be causing the difference (causing the effect). This is a rather long-winded way of saying that inferential statistics are all about identifying whether an effect is significant. Let us look at significance in a little more detail because it is worth understanding this well; after all, it is the main purpose of all inferential statistical procedures to produce the level of significance.

It may come as a surprise to you to hear that statistics never prove anything. It follows that, to a large extent, science doesn't prove anything either. This may seem strange because most of us have a notion of science that has to do with objectivity and facts. After all, surely science is all about the discovery of known things rather than things that are about opinion and belief. In truth, statistics are often at the core of what we know of as science. Science is about teasing out from everything we don't know the one or two things that we might know or that we think we know. Science recognises the world as an uncertain place but tries to tease out which bits of the world we can be more certain about. Statistics deal with this uncertainty by identifying exactly how uncertain we are.

'Probability' is a word that is used to indicate the degree to which we are sure about something. However, probability reflects the fact that we never allow ourselves to be 100% certain about anything. In fact, there are a few things that we think we are certain about; these things are called laws in science. I am as certain as I can be that if I held an apple in my hand and then dropped that apple, it would drop and not float off into the atmosphere. The behaviour of my apple is pretty predictable and is related to Newton's law of gravity. So, we do think we know some things, but there are very few such laws and very few indeed that can be said to relate to healthcare practice.

Theories are a step or two down the knowledge ladder from laws. A theory, such as psychoanalytical or Freudian theory, is a collection of closely interrelated ideas that have some empirical referents, meaning that the theory relates in at least a few ways to what we regard as known facts. However, theory is always evolving. A theory, such as psychoanalytical theory, is in fact a law that is still growing up and still making mistakes.

So, to understand both science and statistical analysis, we must appreciate that the world is a very, very uncertain place. We do know a little about our world, but there is a great deal that we still do not understand. As we apply research to push back the boundaries of knowledge, our ignorance of the world takes the form of apparently chance findings. There are things, or variables, in our world that behave unpredictably, because we don't understand them fully. There are other variables of which we are not yet even aware. These partly or completely unknown variables influence our research. It sometimes seems that as soon as we think we know about variable *a*, variable *b* comes along and proves us wrong. It may even be that we don't know what variable *b* is and that for the moment we have to refer to it as 'chance'. Chance is that part of the world that we do not understand but is still active and may impact on us and on our research.

The world of science is unpredictable and changing. However, we do have a way of measuring the impact of what we don't yet know. It is this that we call 'probability'. The purpose of almost all inferential statistical analyses is the measurement of probability – that is, the measurement of the risk that the effect we are looking at may be caused solely by chance. Probability informs us of the effect that unknown variables (or chance) may be having on our work.

Let us say that we have tested a new analgesic drug against a placebo. We have tested the drug by asking participants to rate their pain after taking the drug or the placebo. We now have one set of data for the placebo and one set of data for the new drug. The two sets of data look different and we suspect that the new drug has worked better than the placebo. However, we need to make sure that our result could not have occurred by chance, so that if we ran the research again we would get a different result, perhaps one that supported the placebo. So, we have run a statistical analysis on the data because we know that this will tell us the probability of the result being due to chance.

Inferential statistical procedures (statistics) are designed to produce a value for probability, which tells us what risk there is that the result of the research was due just to chance. This value is indicated by the letter *P*, followed by a number. Take a look at some examples here:

$P = 0.05$ There is a 5% risk that the result is due only to chance.

$P < 0.001$ There is a less than 1 in 1000 risk that the result is due only to chance.

Both these results could be regarded as significant. The word 'significant' is used when we think it is safe to assume that chance did not play a part in the result of the analysis. However, it is up to us (you and me) to decide what is significant. A probability of 0.05, meaning a risk of 5% (5 in 100), is generally regarded as the minimum level for significance. However, for drug trials, we might want to be much more certain that chance has had no part to play in our research.

Example from practice

Imagine that you are due to drive across a bridge that spans a wide, deep river. You have been told that the bridge is safe. The designers of the bridge are sure about this and their research was significant to $P = 0.05$ (5%).

Would you drive across this bridge? I think that I would want that P to be a much smaller number.

Statistical analysis is a real help in determining the risk that the result of our research is due only to chance. However, it is important that we understand that the calculation of probability, and indeed research and science in general, can never, ever prove anything. We can never, ever be that certain about any of our research. Even if we have a very small P value (as in $P < 0.0000000000001$), there will always be a 1 at the end of the zeros. That 1 is the necessary acceptance that we can never be wholly sure. It is an acceptance that we can be wrong, that we are fallible and ignorant of many of the factors that play a part in what we are seeking to research. Perhaps this is the ultimate irony for the scientific age, for indeed we have demonstrated here that we can never be sure. In searching for truths and facts about our world, we have discovered something quite disturbing – that we can never be sure about anything. This should not worry us too much. Knowing that we are uncertain means that it is important to measure that level of uncertainty in our research – that is what probability does and it is chiefly the reason for us using statistical analysis in the first place.

When your tutor tells you that your essay needs a little more analysis, he or she is really saying that your essay needs a little more of 'you' in it, more of your own thoughts, your effort to make sense of the content that you have found in books and journals. It is just the same with research: the analysis is something that goes on inside the researcher's head. Statistical procedures cannot think; rather, they are tools to help us discern what the data contain. In essence, statistical procedures tell us whether a particular finding (a result) may have occurred by chance or whether it is likely to show a true difference or correlation between groups of data.

Let's look at our imaginary research project on patient pain. Here, we had two groups of patients; both groups had pain. We gave one group an analgesic drug and we used the other group as a control – that is, we didn't give them anything. Let's say that these are the resulting data (pain scores).

Control group	Drug group
1	1
2	2
1	2
2	1
1	2
2	1
1	2
2	1
1	2
2	1
2	2
10	7
10	7
10	7
10	7
10	7
10	7
10	7
10	7
10	7
107 sum	80 sum
5.35 mean	4.0 mean
4.33 standard deviation	2.81 standard deviation
Mann–Whitney test = 159.5 ($P = 0.257$)[1]	

[1] SPSS version 16.

New words

Inferential statistics Statistics used to draw inferences from the data. Inferential statistics are used to give us a measure of significance, to tell us the likelihood that a measured difference (between two groups of data) could have occurred by chance. In contrast, descriptive statistics, such as total and mean, merely describe or summarise the data.

Each patient has scored their pain on a scale of 1-10, with 1 being little or no pain and 10 being a lot of pain. If we look at the average (mean) score for each group, we see that we have a pretty conclusive result in favour of the analgesic group. This seems to show that the patients who received the analgesia experienced less pain:

Control group average pain score = 5.35

Drug group average pain score = 4.0

So there we have it: although we need a larger sample size to be certain of this effect (the result), it looks quite clear that giving people analgesia will reduce their pain. However, let's just look at the other numbers to make sure. The total score (sum) seems to agree with the mean scores: the control group scored higher (had more pain) than the drug group (had less pain). Now let's look at the standard deviation. This is a measure of the dispersion around the mean. This is nothing more than a technical term for how spread out the values are. Note that the standard deviation for the control group is quite large, meaning that the data are quite spread out around the mean. Look at the data for the control group: some scores are low, while others are high. The average value is 5.35; what do you think about this?

- Do we expect the mean to reflect or summarise the data?

- In this case, does the mean accurately reflect the data?

- Did any single participant (patient) give a score on or near 5.35?

The mean should reflect the data, but here it doesn't. The mean does not reflect the data because the data vary a lot. In fact, there seem to be two groups of patients in the control group - some have a lot of pain and some don't seem to have much pain. Their pain scores vary a lot - in other words, there is a high level of dispersion around the mean and, consequently, the standard deviation (which measures the dispersion around the mean) is relatively high for the control group.

Now let's look at the result for the Mann-Whitney test. This is an inferential statistical procedure, designed to show whether the difference between two groups of data could have occurred only by chance – that is, had nothing to do with whether the patients were given analgesia or not. The result from the Mann-Whitney test is 0.257. To be considered significant (not due to chance), the result would have to be less than (<) 0.05. The number we have (0.257) is much bigger than (>) 0.05. So, there is a difference between the scores given by the two groups of patients, but that difference is not significant. In other words, we have no reason to believe that the difference as represented by the mean values was related to the use or otherwise of the analgesic drug.

The Mann-Whitney procedure does what most inferential statistical procedures do: it measures the variance *within* each group of data and then it measures the variance *between* the (two) groups of data. In general:

> If the *between groups* variance (difference between the groups of data) is greater than the *within groups* variance, then the result will be significant.

> If the *between groups* variance (difference between the groups of data) is less than the *within groups* variance, then the result will be non-significant.

So, statistical procedures tell us whether a difference that exists (between two or more groups of data) is likely to be due to a chance event or to the thing that we are trying to measure.

What statistical procedures tell us about data is actually quite limited. We need to be careful how we use and how we interpret the results of statistical procedures. All the time, we need to engage our mind when looking at data and the results of any statistical analysis. Indeed, if you look at the data in our example again, you will immediately spot the problem. It is now obvious that the variation in scores within each of the two groups is not expected and this warns us that something is wrong. You have learned a lot. Now you can look at data and provide at least an educated guess at whether the result will be significant or not. Know about statistics? You already know them so well that you can anticipate what the result will be.

Using the right statistical procedure

There are a lot of statistical procedures (you may know them as statistical tests). Some procedures are appropriate in some situations and some in other situations. So, the first thing we need to know is how to choose the most appropriate statistical procedure.

New words

Correlation The word 'correlation' is similar to 'association'. We deal in correlations when we want to know whether one set of data behaves synchronously with another. Children's weights and ages do this. There are lightweight older children and heavyweight younger children but, on the whole, as children grow older (one set of data) their weight increases (another set of data). In determining this, we do not conclude that weight and age are the same thing; they are not the same thing but these two different things (variables) are correlated.

The fact that two sets of data are correlated does not mean that one variable causes the other. Weight is associated with age but being heavy does not cause one to be old.

If you are reading a research paper, you will want to check that the statistical procedures that were used were the appropriate ones. However, there is an important caveat here. If you have selected your research paper from a good-quality journal, then the paper will have been peer-reviewed. In this way, it will have been checked by someone who does not know the author. The person who did this checking will have more knowledge of statistical analysis than you are likely to have. So, what does this mean? In practice, it means that you can be fairly sure that the proper analyses were conducted and that you only really need to document (in your essay) why it was appropriate.

So, what do you need to know? It would be useful for you to know a little about how statistical procedures are chosen, so let us look at a small range of commonly used statistical procedures.

Correlations or differences?

There are two fundamentally different questions that we can ask of data: are groups of data correlated or are they different? Remember: we have to be clear and focused about what we are looking for in the data. Sometimes we want to find out whether one group of data correlates with another group of data, and sometimes we want to find out whether one group of data is different from another group of data.

We might want to know whether children's weight is correlated with their age. Of course, children's weight *does* correlate with their age. As children grow older, their weight tends to increase. This stands to reason, doesn't it? This is an important point: whatever analysis we choose should be logically derived from what we want to find out; indeed, it should always stand to reason in this way. Would we want to know whether children's weight is different from their age? No, such a question does not make sense. The questions we ask of the data should always make sense. This is always sense that absolutely anyone can understand.

Now let us think about the other main question we can ask of data: is one group of data different from another?

Let us assume that we have a sample of patients who are all in pain. We divide this sample into two groups. We give one group an analgesic drug and the other group we give no intervention.

We then ask the whole sample to tell us how much pain they have. Do we want to find out whether the two sets of data (the pain scores) are correlated? No, of course not; we want to know whether the two sets of data are different. This is often the question asked of experiments – that is, does the experimental variable (the intervention) cause an effect on the dependent variable (the pain score)?

We need to note here that different statistical procedures are used where we look for evidence of correlations and where we look for evidence of differences. We will look at some of these procedures later in this chapter, but for now let's just note that correlations and differences relate to one of the important ways in which we look at data.

Identifying the correct statistical tool: key questions to ask

New words

Univariate With one variable; for example, the effect of providing analgesia on pain perception.

Multivariate With more than one variable; for example, the effect of providing (a) an analgesic drug and (b) psychological therapy on (a) pain, (b) anxiety and (c) contentedness with treatment.

How many groups are contained in the analysis?

It is easiest to think about data analysis as just involving two groups of data. In fact, all researchers would probably like to keep to just two groups. Unfortunately, it is sometimes necessary to analyse data from more than two groups at the same time. For example, we might need to compare the effect of two analgesic drugs against a control; this would give us three groups of data. Sometimes, we know that there are lots of variables that might be causing an effect and so we need to include them all in the analysis.

There are two important considerations here. The first is that the number of groups of data will help to determine which statistical procedure we use. The second is that statistical analyses become more complex as the number of groups of data increases. No one wants this to happen; it is seriously undesirable. An analysis should always teach us something new about the data; it should never confuse us. Laboratory researchers will go to great lengths to reduce the number of variables with which they have to deal at any one time. They will ensure that they have only one chemical in their test tube and not a mix of chemicals. Unfortunately, those of us who wish to research human beings often find that we can't squash them into test tubes: they usually won't fit and they are rarely willing to be put in one anyway. All too often, we are interested in the complex mix of variables that is human life, and so our analyses tend to be multivariate, composed of several, or even many, variables.

We need to be clear about the relationship between a 'group' of data and 'variables'. We already know that there are two broad categories of variable; that is, 'independent variable' and 'dependent variable'. The independent variable might be 'treatment type' and the dependent variable might be 'recorded pain level'. However, although this study might have only one independent variable ('treatment type'), this might be divided into three groups, or 'conditions' (when these are categories, they are sometimes called 'factors'). These conditions might be 'drug A', 'drug B' and 'control' (no drug). So, here we have one independent variable with three groups (three conditions). These three 'parts' of the independent variable are going to produce three sets of data (groups of data).

A study might have more than one independent variable (each with its own conditions or groups) and it might have more than one dependent variable. We might, for example, want to measure the effect of two independent variables, 'treatment type' and 'sex', on two dependent variables, 'recorded pain' and 'days in hospital'. We might want to do this because we think there might be an interaction between these variables. Let's put this graphically:

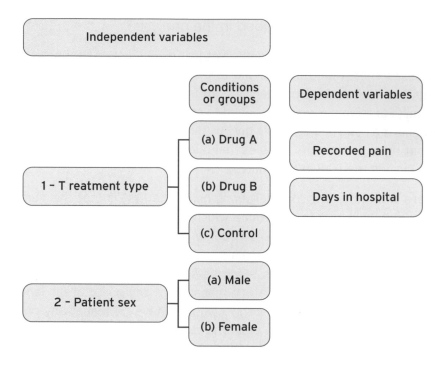

Correlation studies do not (really) have an independent or dependent variable – they just have two variables. We might want to see if child age and child height correlate, for example. Age and height are not usefully categorised as independent or dependent variables. Sometimes, however, we will need to identify what are the independent variable(s), how many conditions each individual independent variable has and how many dependent variables there are. This will be necessary if we are to be able to select an appropriate statistical analysis for our study design.

What is the level of measurement?

This is easy: we have already worked it out. We have noted that numerical data exist within one of three levels of measurement. We noted that each of these levels of measurement has a separate collection of statistical procedures associated with it. These are:

- nominal (categories);

- ordinal (items placed in order or any short scale);

- interval or ratio[2] (a long scale).

[2] When it comes to numerical analysis, interval and ratio data are treated similarly.

Is the design related or unrelated?

This is the last question we need to ask, at least for the range of statistical procedures that we will be looking at here. A related design is one where the data are collected from the same sample of people (here, we are usually dealing with people) on more than one occasion. So, it will be clear now that an unrelated design is where the researcher collects data from two or more different groups of people. We do not need to ask this question when correlations are being looked for because correlational designs are always related and, in any case, they have their own range of statistical procedures.

It is probably the case that more research designs in healthcare are of the unrelated kind. When we determined the effect of providing an analgesic to patients in pain, we had two groups; one group was given an analgesic drug and the other was not provided with any intervention. Those two groups of people were different people; they didn't even know each other. If we had used a before-after design, we might have put both groups of people together and then measured their pain before and after giving them (all) the analgesic drug. In this last situation, we would have a related design.

Related designs tend to be longitudinal in quality, with data being collected from the same people on more than one occasion. With unrelated designs, data are collected from two or more different groups of people at more or less the same time.

You can now select the appropriate statistical procedure

It will have occurred to you by now that we have been looking at statistics without actually mentioning many of them by name. This is because statistical procedures all do pretty much the same job, but there are different procedures (different statistics) for different kinds of data and where we want to ask different questions about the data; for example, whether the data contain correlations or differences.

With the help of Figure 6.1, you are now able to select the appropriate statistical procedure for a range of commonly used research designs. Even if some of this chapter has been a little difficult to grasp, you do now have the skills to select the right statistical procedure from quite a range of statistics that will fill a whole page. Take a quick look at Figure 6.1, be suitably awestruck and then read on to discover that you already do understand how to select the right statistical procedure for a variety of research designs.

In 1 minute you will have:

- been horrified by the number of statistical procedures available;
- decided that it is too complex for anyone to understand.

In 2 more minutes you will have:

- demonstrated to yourself that you do understand it and that you can select appropriate statistical procedures for a variety of research designs.

Now look at Figure 6.1 and select the most appropriate statistical procedure for the following research designs.

Design 1

This study looks at the difference in regard for the NHS between a sample of people aged 20–30 years and a sample of people aged 65–85 years. The participants are asked 'Do you trust the NHS to care for you when you are ill?' The participants are asked to answer simply 'yes', 'no' or 'not sure'.

The data produced by this study are *nominal* (the categories are 'yes', 'no' and 'not sure').

It is hypothesised that there will be *differences* between the responses from the younger and the older group of participants.

The design is *unrelated* because the two groups of participants have nothing to do with each other (the design would be related if the study asked younger people about the NHS and then waited until years later, when they had aged and become older people, before asking them the same question again).

Common statistical procedure

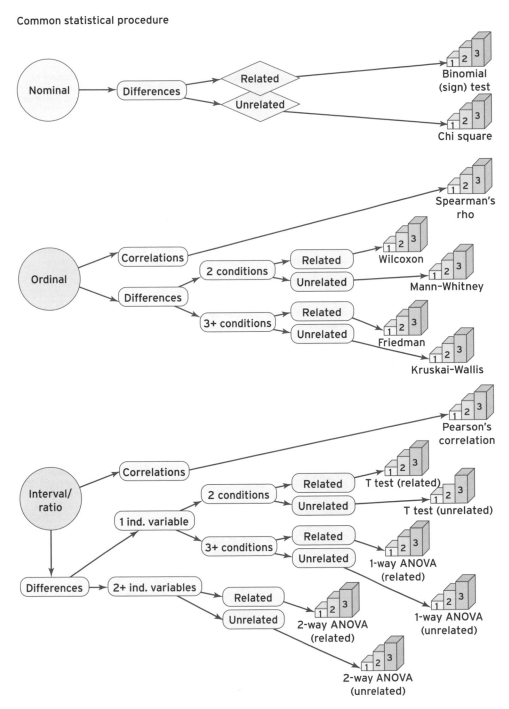

Figure 6.1 Selecting the appropriate statistical procedure.

Statistics for nominal data

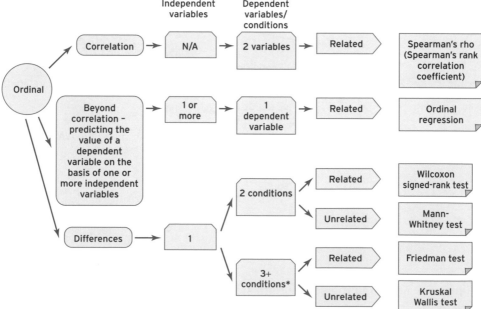

* 'Association' is a kind of middle term between 'differences' and 'correlation' but which doesn't quite mean 'correlation'. It is commonly used for 'differences' but is also used where the lack of 'difference' can be meaningful (association). Phi and Cramér's V are specifically used to measure whether one variable is 'associated' with another variable. chi square itself is chiefly used where 'differences' are expected.
In practice, chi square, phi and Cramér's V tend to be calculated at the same time.

** The independent variable (sometimes here called a 'predictor variable') can be either nominal data or may exist as a scale. The dependent variable in logistic regression will be nominal (categories).

Non-parametric statistics for ordinal data

* Three or more different groups for an unrelated design, or one group measured on three or more occasions for a related design. Related designs are sometimes referred to as 'repeated measures'.

Parametric statistics for interval and ratio data: correlations and predictions

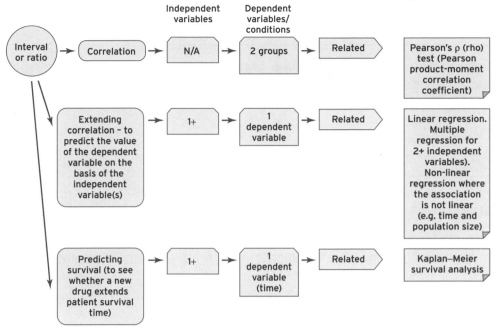

Parametric statistics for interval and ratio data: differences

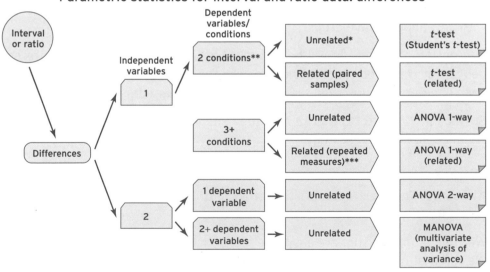

* Unrelated, sometimes referred to as 'unpaired' or 'independent' samples.

** Two groups, or, for a related design, one group measured on two occasions.

*** For a related design, the independent variable is often 'time'. The dependent variables are measures taken from one group (one sample) taken on three or more occasions.

Look at Figure 6.1 and write here the name of the statistical procedure that should be used for this study:

_____

Correct! You did it: it is chi square. Let's do that again with something much more complicated (I am sure you will get this right too).

Design 2

We want to run an experiment to see whether anti-hypertensive drugs, increased exercise or both anti-hypertensive drugs and increased exercise have the best effect on the blood pressure of people being treated for hypertension.

The data collected by the study will be blood pressure recordings. Blood pressure will be measured in mmHg on a scale that (theoretically) can be zero (or less) and that is continuous (it is possible to have a systolic BP of 120.3456 mmHg, should we wish for that degree of accuracy). So the level of measurement is *interval/ratio*.

The study hypothesises that there will be *differences* between the data collected from the three groups of patients.

In this experiment, there is *one independent variable* – the type of treatment. This independent variable has *three conditions* – the three groups of patients, i.e. anti-hypertensive drugs, increased exercise and increased exercise together with anti-hypertensive drugs.

The design of the study will be *unrelated* because we will be using different people for the three conditions (if we used the same people, exposing them to each condition in turn, then the design would be related).

So, look at Figure 6.1 and write here the name of the statistical procedure that should be used for this study:

_____

Awesome! The most appropriate statistical procedure is the one-way ANOVA (unrelated).

Well done! So, statistics are easy. The research design tells us which one to use. We run that one-way analysis of variance (unrelated) in a statistics application such as SPSS® just like we use a word processor to process words.

In 1 minute you have:

- been horrified by the number of statistical procedures available; ✓ ?
- decided that it is too complex for anyone to understand. ✓ ?

In 2 more minutes you have:

- proved to yourself that you do understand it and that you can select appropriate statistical procedures for a variety of research designs. ✓ ?

What does a one-way analysis of variance do? It does what all inferential statistical procedures do: it looks at whether the within group variance is greater or less than the between group variance (whether the difference in BP scores *between* the three groups of hypertensive patients is greater or less than the degree to which the scores *within* each group vary). In doing this, it will tell us to what degree we can be sure that any difference between the groups is caused by the effect of the independent variable or whether we should deduce that any such difference is due merely to chance. The one-way analysis of variance will give us a probability value (P), which will tell us what risk there is that any difference between the groups is due just to chance. If you understand the meaning of the P value in a one-way analysis of variance, you understand its meaning in all inferential statistical procedures.

A real example from the literature: data analysis using Pearson chi square

Yildirim *et al.* (2010) used Pearson chi square to determine whether there was a difference between medical and nursing students in relation to their perception of the usefulness of complementary and alternative medicine. If you have access to an online full text database or to the *Journal of Clinical Nursing*, you should be able to get a copy of this article:

Yildirim, Y., S. Parlar *et al.* (2010). 'An analysis of nursing and medical students' attitudes towards and knowledge of complementary and alternative medicine (CAM)'. *Journal of Clinical Nursing* 19(7–8): 1157–1166.

General attitudes about complementary and alternative medicine (CAM) of nursing and medical students (% of respondents)

	Nursing students			Medical students			
	Agree	Undecided	Don't agree	Agree	Undecided	Don't agree	p-value*
	%	%	%	%	%	%	
CAM practices should be integrated in my School's curriculum (n = 969)	61.3	23.4	15.4	37.9	22.3	39.3	<0.001
CAM practices should be included in clinical care (n = 969)	57.8	24.9	17.3	32.6	22.9	44.5	<0.001
CAM is a threat to public health (n = 970)	10.3	25.4	64.3	20.4	36.8	42.7	<0.001
CAM therapies not tested in a scientific manner should be discouraged (n = 971)	64.4	17.6	18.0	77.5	8.5	14.0	<0.001
The results of CAM are in most cases due to a placebo effect (n = 967)	38.8	38.3	22.9	47.5	32.3	20.2	<0.05
CAM therapies stimulated the natural therapeutic power of the body (n = 969)	62.9	28.4	8.6	51.4	38.3	9.5	<0.01

*Pearson chi-square test was used to determine the differences between nursing and medical students.

This table is taken from page 1160 of the article. Yildirim *et al.* simply asked nurses and medical students questions about their impression of the usefulness of complementary and alternative medicine (CAM). The responses were categorised as 'agree', 'undecided' and 'don't agree'. So, the data elicited from the participants was 'nominal'; that is, they existed as 'categories'. If we look at the first line of results in the above table, we can see that they form a 2×3 grid which looks like this:

Analysis – CAM practices should be integrated in my school curriculum

	Agree	Undecided	Don't agree	Pearson chi square
Nursing students	61.3	23.4	15.4	
Medical students	37.9	22.3	39.3	(*P* < 0.001)

Don't worry about the chi square statistic for the moment. Just look at the figures; that is, 'eyeball' them. When I look at them, I can see that nursing students were more likely to agree that CAM should be taught to students than were medical students. However, to convince others of this result, the researchers needed to demonstrate that it was unlikely to have occurred by chance. To do this, they subjected the numbers in this 2 × 3 grid to statistical analysis using Pearson chi square. The result ($P < 0.001$) indicated that the risk of this result being due to chance alone was less than 1:1000. We can therefore be reasonably certain that the result that we can see in this grid of numbers was in fact caused by what we think caused it; that is, a difference between nursing and medical students on the value of complementary and alternative medicine in the curriculum.

Statistical procedures used in Cochrane systematic reviews

Systematic reviews look at all the research on a particular focus. In this, they are similar to literature reviews. However, systematic reviews go much further in that they collect all the data from the range of studies reviewed. The data is then put together and analysed; this is generally referred to as 'meta-analysis'. This process can identify those studies that add most to the analysis and those that do not. In practice, this deals effectively with the problem of two (or more) studies having conflicting findings. The statistical tests used in systematic reviews are presented in a rather unique, graphical format. This is designed to make the statistical analysis easier to understand. Here is a typical example from a systematic review by Derry *et al.* (2012).

Review: Caffeine as an analgesic adjuvant for acute pain in adults
Comparison: 1 Analgesic plus caffeine versus analgesic alone by pain condition
Outcome: 1 At least 50% of maximum pain relief

Study or subgroup	Analgesic + caffeine n/N	Analgesic n/N	Risk Ratio M-H,Fixed,95% CI	Weight	Risk Ratio M-H,Fixed,95% CI
1 Headache					
Diamond 2000	65/97	55/99		3.4 %	1.21 [0.96, 1.51]
Diener 2005	429/482	418/498		25.8 %	1.06 [1.01, 1.11]
Migliardi 1994	253/336	221/332		14.0 %	1.13 [1.03, 1.25]
Migliardi 1994	258/339	229/337		14.4 %	1.12 [1.02, 1.23]
Subtotal (95% CI)	**1254**	**1266**		**57.6 %**	**1.10 [1.06, 1.15]**

Total events: 1005 (Analgesic + caffeine), 923 (Analgesic)
Heterogeneity: Chi² = 3.26, df = 3 (P = 0.35); I² =8%
Test for overall effect: Z = 4.43 (P < 0.00001)

2 Dysmenorrhoea					
Ali 2007	134/310	121/310		7.6 %	1.11 [0.92, 1.34]
Subtotal (95% CI)	**310**	**310**		**7.6 %**	**1.11 [0.92, 1.34]**

Total events: 134 (Analgesic + caffeine), 121 (Analgesic)
Heterogeneity: not applicable
Test for overall effect: Z = 1.06 (P = 0.29)

3 Postoperative/postpartum					
Forbes 1990	17/66	17/68		1.1 %	1.03 [0.58, 1.84]
Forbes 1991	24/44	17/48		1.0 %	1.54 [0.96, 2.46]
Forbes 1991	19/49	13/49		0.8 %	1.46 [0.82, 2.62]
Laska 1983	57/80	56/81		3.5 %	1.03 [0.84, 1.26]
Laska 1983	39/62	42/68		2.5 %	1.02 [0.78, 1.33]
Laska 1983	42/45	37/46		2.3 %	1.16 [0.99, 1.37]
Laska 1983	32/56	26/54		1.7 %	1.19 [0.83, 1.70]
Laska 1983	42/57	28/50		1.9 %	1.32 [0.98, 1.76]
Laska 1983	51/80	47/81		2.9 %	1.10 [0.86, 1.41]
Laska 1983	34/40	33/42		2.0 %	1.08 [0.88, 1.33]
Laska 1983	38/62	40/68		2.4 %	1.04 [0.79, 1.38]
Laska 1983	50/78	52/81		3.2 %	1.00 [0.79, 1.26]
Laska 1983	45/64	43/66		2.7 %	1.08 [0.85, 1.37]
Laska 1983	42/56	38/60		2.3 %	1.18 [0.93, 1.51]
McQuay 1996 (1)	34/89	2/31		0.2 %	5.92 [1.51, 23.22]
Sunshine 1996	36/50	33/50		2.1 %	1.09 [0.84, 1.42]
Sunshine 1996	24/50	17/51		1.1 %	1.44 [0.89, 2.34]
Winter 1983	19/40	20/41		1.2 %	0.97 [0.62, 1.53]
Subtotal (95% CI)	**1068**	**1035**		**34.8 %**	**1.15 [1.07, 1.23]**

Total events: 645 (Analgesic + caffeine), 561 (Analgesic)
Heterogeneity: Chi² = 14.67, df = 17 (P = 0.62); I² =0.0%
Test for overall effect: Z = 3.78 (P = 0.00016)

| **Total (95% CI)** | **2632** | **2611** | | **100.0 %** | **1.12 [1.08, 1.16]** |

Total events: 1784 (Analgesic + caffeine), 1605 (Analgesic)
Heterogeneity: Chi² = 18.83, df = 22 (P = 0.66); I² =0.0%
Test for overall effect: Z = 5.77 (P < 0.00001)
Test for subgroup differences: Chi² = 0.93, df = 2 (P = 0.63), I² =0.0%

```
        0.2    0.5    1    2    5
     Favours A            Favours A + C
```

(1) 3 doses of caffeine combined

You may have wondered why pharmaceutical companies often put caffeine into analgesic medicines. We can see here evidence that caffeine is effective in enhancing the analgesic properties of paracetamol and ibuprofen when taken for headache and postoperative pain. At first sight, this chart looks confusing, so let's look at it in more detail.

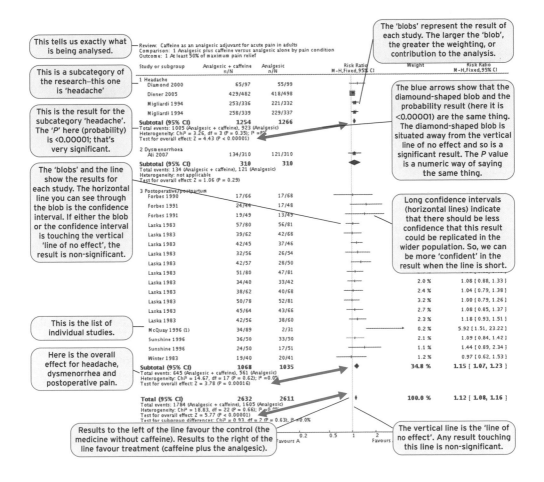

The statistics used in Cochrane reviews are based on 'odds ratios' (similar to the statistical procedures used in horse-racing). We use the word 'odds' when we say 'What are the odds that this horse will win the race?' The actual statistic used in this analysis (above) is called the 'risk ratio' and is used when the data are continuous (interval or ratio data). However, the really good thing about Cochrane charts is that the chart will look the same whatever statistical procedure has been used.

Cochrane charts (sometimes loosely called 'odds ratio charts') always have a vertical line (the line of no effect) with 'blobs' shown on one or other side of the line. One side of the line is designated the 'control' and the other side is designated the 'treatment (intervention)'. In this way, a result (a blob) will do one of three things.

1. It will sit in the control area, showing that the result supports the control (often a placebo) or 'normal care'.

2. It will sit in the treatment area, showing that the result supports the intervention. In the example here, the 'treatment' is the use of caffeine together with the analgesic.

3. It will sit on or touch the vertical line of no effect, or the blob's confidence interval (the horizontal line that goes through the blob) will touch the line of no effect. This means that there is 'no effect'. The result of the study neither supports the intervention nor the control.

You can see from the chart that each study has its own result, and we can see each result in relation to the other results. However, you will also see that there is a summary result and the summary results are diamond-shaped. In this way, Cochrane charts show us a meta-analysis of all the results, together with one final summary result. The meta-analysis is a way of dealing with conflicting results. The analysis does not just calculate an average score from all the individual ones; rather, the process works out the contribution that each study made to the analysis, called the 'weighting'. We can see the weighting for each study, reflected in the size of the blob. Studies that were able to contribute more, perhaps because they had a larger sample size or a clearer 'result', have a bigger input into the summary result. In this way, the meta-analysis used in Cochrane systematic reviews is an effective way of summarising many individual studies, concluding with one single summary measure which can always be seen to: (1) support the control; (2) support the intervention; or (3) show no effect at all.

Concluding remarks

Data analysis of any kind exists to serve two purposes. The first purpose of analysis is to discover things (effects) within the data, effects that might not be at all obvious from looking at the raw data (sometimes called 'eyeballing the data'). This is exactly the same mechanism that you employ when you apply analysis to the discussion in your essay. The second purpose is to summarise the data to make them more understandable and to make it possible to communicate them in a way that will be both succinct and meaningful. However, even the most complex statistical analysis is only a tool. Analysis does not remove from the researcher the responsibility to consider the data carefully and to evaluate critically what the analysis has shown, together with any weaknesses inherent in that analysis. As professionals who may be asked to integrate research findings into practice, healthcare practitioners are free to criticise an analysis and to suggest alternative interpretations of the data.

Data analysis, especially when it is quantitative and statistical, probably does scare many people away from research. However, we have seen here that data analysis really can be easy to understand. We should bear in mind that no one knows everything about data analysis and that even the most accomplished researchers tend to be familiar only with the kinds of analysis used in their own field of work. Of course, there are many forms of data analysis that have not been covered in this chapter, but the principles of data analysis, as those principles affect almost any kind of data, have indeed been covered here. That's a great start and one that will allow you to develop your understanding further.

Summary

- A knowledge of mathematics is not needed. Researchers use computer applications, not a pencil and paper.

- Inferential statistical procedures (tests) do not prove anything; rather, they demonstrate the degree to which chance may have had an effect on the research.

- It is up to you and me to decide whether the level of probability (as in $P = 0.05$) is acceptable. We are free to suggest that a higher level of significance would be desirable.

- Selecting the correct statistical procedure is not usually difficult, even though there are many statistical procedures available.

- In general, the purpose of any analysis is to summarise the data and to extract from the data information that is often not otherwise readily apparent.

Further reading

A great way to learn more about statistical analysis is to explore the computer application known as SPSS. This is an expensive product, but most universities make it available to students. SPSS originally stood for Statistical Package for the Social Sciences. More information on the SPSS suite of applications can be found at **www.spss.com.**

SPSS is shipped with some example data files; your university computer centre will show you where to find these. Try loading in some data and simply play with the application.

There are several good books that can help you to get to grips with SPSS and with quantitative data analysis, including these:

Pallant, J. (2007). *SPSS Survival Manual: A Step by Step Guide to Data Analysis Using SPSS for Windows*. Milton Keynes: Open University Press.

Field, A. (2005). *Discovering Statistics Using SPSS*. London: Sage Publications Limited.

References

Derry, C. J., S. Derry *et al.* (2012) 'Caffeine as an analgesic adjuvant for acute pain in adults'. *Cochrane Database of Systematic Reviews* DOI: 10.1002/14651858. CD009281.pub2.

Yildirim, Y., S. Parlar *et al.* (2010). 'An analysis of nursing and medical students' attitudes towards and knowledge of complementary and alternative medicine (CAM)'. *Journal of Clinical Nursing* 19(7-8): 1157-1166.

Chapter 7
Qualitative research – what exactly is it?

CHAPTER OBJECTIVES

The objectives for this chapter are to:

- Define qualitative research

- Explain how the subjectivity of qualitative research can be seen positively

- Introduce ethnography, phenomenology and grounded theory.

Chapter outline

This chapter will introduce qualitative research, both its 'methodological' traditions and its practice. At first sight, qualitative research can seem a lot easier to understand than its quantitative sibling. Qualitative research papers are written in easy-to-understand English, they have a 'friendlier' style and describe their research without (usually) using any statistics at all. However, qualitative research can lure the new researcher into a false sense of security. The 'results' of qualitative studies are, indeed, easy to understand but how those results were obtained is not at all straightforward. Let me guess, in fact, that there were two subjects you never really liked at school or university. My guess is that one of those subjects will have been maths and the other will have been 'philosophy'. In this chapter we shall leave maths and statistics behind, only to fall into a dark and muddy pit full of philosophy. Do not despair! You have got this far with your sanity intact and you will succeed with this chapter too.

In previous chapters, we dealt with statistics in the same pragmatic manner that healthcare practitioners deal with most things. We found that we could understand statistics and their use without having to wallow in any mathematical theory. In this chapter, we will examine qualitative research without having to become philosophers first. Qualitative research is an inherently practical and pragmatic undertaking (ask any PhD student). It must then be the case that even the muddiest recesses of qualitative methodology can be seen in ways that are practical and pragmatic; in this chapter, we will be seeing things in just this way.

Words – reminder

Quantitative research Quantitative research usually deals with numbers and is designed to test an idea, a hypothesis or a theory (quantitative research is 'deductive'). We think, for example, that drug A is effective because drugs that are similar to drug A are known to be effective. However, we need to determine its effectiveness, and in a way that will convince everybody.

Qualitative research Qualitative research usually deals with spoken or written language. Qualitative research usually starts with a question like 'How do people experience this particular health problem?' In this way, qualitative research explores a phenomenon from a starting position that is assumed to be one of ignorance. That starting point is the question itself, not a theory or an already assumed knowledge base (it is 'inductive'). Qualitative research is used when we know so little about a human experience that we do not know exactly what questions to ask.

New words

Inductive research From data to theory. The researcher starts with an acknowledgement that little or nothing is known about the human experience in question. Data collected and analysed elicit themes, constructs or theory which can then be used to describe or explain the experience.

Deductive research From theory to data. Often used in psychological research. The researcher starts with preconceived ideas of what the data will be like. Such research starts with a hypothesis or the research is carried out within a theoretical model, as in researching an aspect of Freudian theory.

What is qualitative research?

> Qualitative research explores the social world from the perspective of participants. It is characterized by an emphasis on understanding other persons' perspectives and their experiences, and the interpretations and meanings they bring and give to events and situations.
>
> *(Astin and Long 2009, p. 390)*

> '. . . it is the method of choice to understand the complexities of being human'
>
> *(Frank and Polkinghorne 2010, p. 52)*

Those looking at research for the first time are often put off by the apparent complexity of quantitative research. When they stumble across qualitative research they think that they have found a much more 'approachable' form of research. Qualitative research rarely uses numbers or statistics; instead, the results are reported in textual form, often in a manner that can be readily understood. Qualitative researchers usually reject the passive voice in their writing and are happy to refer to themselves as 'I' and to refer to participants by (fictitious) first names. This alone makes reading the text a much more 'human' experience. Indeed, qualitative research does seem to be in touch with the feminine side of human nature. It seems to exist in a 'softer' and more 'sensitive' contrast to what Nicholls (2009a, p. 529) refers to as the 'andro-centric' nature of quantitative research.

So it is a little perverse that qualitative research can be quite difficult to do. Its methodology is tied up with some very complex philosophical ideas and it is also the case that data collection and analysis can take a considerable amount of time. One should not adopt qualitative research out of a mistaken belief that it is 'easier'; nothing could be further from the truth. In any case, neither quantitative nor qualitative research should be adopted for any other reason than that they are the right choice for what the researcher is trying to find out. Quantitative and qualitative approaches do not compete with each other; rather, they should be seen as complementary – two different approaches that are available to the questioning practitioner.

Qualitative research is sometimes criticised for being too subjective (Porter 2007). However, this subjectivity is an intentional aspect of qualitative research and is not some kind of flaw in the methodology. Qualitative research is designed to deal with the subjective world and it elects to view that world subjectively. It might be worth a couple of minutes to look at the converse argument, that quantitative research is too objective.

Quantitative research is closely aligned to the notion of 'science' and of the world being an objective and measurable place; this is sometimes called the 'positivist' view of the world. There are certainly aspects of the world that are measurable. We can measure body temperature, for example; this gives us a number (37°C). This number is meaningful to us; we can compare it to other people's body temperature. Values such as body temperature have a consistent nature and are reliable. So, let us be clear, an objective world does exist and quantitative research is well placed to measure it.

Klopper (2008) suggests that we should use qualitative research when:

- there is little known about a topic;

- the research context is poorly understood;

- the boundaries of a domain are poorly understood;

- the phenomenon in question is not quantifiable.

Reflection point

Pause for a while to reflect on what 'science' means to you. Pretend you are lying on the psychiatrist's couch and you are asked to think of words relating to 'science'.

I came up with 'laboratory', 'Bunsen burner', 'lab coat' and 'safety glasses'.

Medicine claims to be a science – the next time you visit your GP, why not ask to be shown his/her laboratory (the word 'laboratory' has to be pronounced with a Germanic or Russian accent). You may, then, be surprised that your GP doesn't actually have one. So how can medicine be a science? If medicine is really a science, medics must be 'scientists' and scientists surely must have a laboratory.

Now take yourself to the main entrance of your university and look at the signpost there. You will probably see directions to the Faculty of Arts and the Faculty of Science. Now ask yourself, 'What is the difference between the two?' It must be a big difference for every university to be divided into arts and science.

That's right, the Faculty of Science has a laboratory and the Faculty of Arts does not (we were right about the laboratory). But can the existence of Bunsen burners and lab coats really be the defining characteristic of science?

Perhaps science deals with facts and art doesn't. No facts in arts then. Perhaps science is objective and methodological. So people who study history and

English literature don't deal in facts and go about their study in a more or less random and uncoordinated way. In fact, both history and English are studied methodologically; facts are dealt with and it is possible to do a PhD and to research both history and English literature.

So what is 'science'? Perhaps it is nothing but an overarching construct with no truly objective meaning - a bit like 'love' and 'God'. Perhaps 'science' does not exist at all.

The problem comes when we begin to think that everything that matters is measurable. The behaviourists in the early 20th century thought, for example, that it would ultimately be possible to know exactly how to bring up children (see Watson 1928; Hardyment 1995). I suspect that most of us who have tried to bring up children are aware that the very complexity and individuality of children makes it impossible to see them objectively as simply a collection of facts and figures. Children, like all human beings, are hopelessly complex, variable and inconsistent. You will recall from your own childhood that you would be well behaved and compliant one day and a true monster the next. We are simply not reliable and we are so complex that even our parents never really get to understand us. In fact, most people would probably claim that they do not even fully understand themselves. This is a real problem for both science and quantitative research, which can only deal with an objective, measurable and consistent world. In fact, the whole point of statistical analysis, so much a central part of quantitative research, is to determine the likelihood that the results obtained might or might not have occurred by chance. To the quantitative researcher, 'chance' is that part of the world that is not yet understood and which may therefore vary and change in ways that are unpredictable. Quantitative researchers aim to design their studies so that 'chance' is kept out of their data. It follows that quantitative research has a real problem when 'everything' is unpredictable (like people).

So science and quantitative research have a problem with phenomena (things) that are inconsistent or unreliable, and that can't be measured with numbers. Now this is not a problem as long as healthcare practitioners only deal in an objective, measurable world. We have no problem with body temperature, the size of an infant's heart shown on a radiograph or a blood count showing anaemia - all these are measurable and reliable indices of an objective world.

The trouble is that healthcare practitioners spend at least part of their time with something that is not objective, is often too complex to measure and too poorly reliable and consistent, something that is often very poorly understood – the person, patient, client: the human being. So it is that healthcare practitioners find themselves asking such questions as:

- What is it like for a patient to experience my operating theatre?

- What sense do young children make of the physiotherapy I provide?

- What is it like to have schizophrenia?

- What meaning do dying people find in a largely secular health service?

In other words, we often want to know about human experience. Here it is that qualitative research has a useful role. In these situations, we cannot give people a questionnaire because we don't know what questions to ask. Instead, what we have to do is ask questions that are little more than prompts, such as 'Tell me what it is like to have schizophrenia.'

Qualitative researchers sometimes talk of human experience yielding 'deep' or 'information-rich' data. Human experience exists as a complex 'weave' of interrelating experiences, all of which are understood in different ways and at different levels, with our understanding of our experiences changing over time. In this way, human experience is not one reality but a 'multiplicity of realities' (Campbell and Roden 2010, p. 114). Furthermore, there are a number of ways of interpreting this reality; context is important. We see things differently in different contexts and our experiences change over time (see the reflection point below).

As healthcare practitioners, we deal with people first and with thermometers second. We are interested in how our patients and clients feel, what it is that they are experiencing. We are interested in these things because we care about people; we want to know how they feel so that we may better help them. It is in these situations that qualitative research has a part to play. In this, it deals with some of the more central and important questions about healthcare and about people's experience of healthcare and of illness and trauma. Qualitative research is 'inductive'. This means that we start from an acknowledged position of ignorance rather than from a pre-existing understanding. Klopper (2008) suggests that inductive research starts with an acknowledgement that we do not know about the phenomenon in question. Nicholls (2009b, p. 587) suggests that '...humans are self-determining. This means that each of us interprets our world in our own unique way, and what comes to be considered "real" is entirely idiosyncratic'. Quantitative research and traditional science simply can't deal with phenomena such as this – qualitative research can.

You know what a policeman is. There is an objective (positivist) truth about policemen. They exist, we can count them; we can measure their height and the size of their feet and plot these on a chart. Policemen exist in the positivist world and we all know that. We all know what a policeman is. We know what their role is. We can hypothesise (deductively) that good citizens will view policemen differently to criminals. These are fixed and unchanging facts (truths) about policemen.

1. Someone has just run into the back of your car. You are not physically hurt but you are shaken by the incident. You are alone and you don't want to talk with the other driver because you are afraid that he might be aggressive. Fortunately, a police car stops close by. The policeman comes over to you and you sense the reassuring calm of someone in authority taking over the situation. He checks you are okay and then goes over to speak to the other driver. In that moment and in that space you view the police very positively.

2. You have spent the day shopping. You are very tired and you are looking forward to going home. You return to the car to find a parking ticket on the windscreen. In the distance, you see a policeman checking parked cars. You find yourself thinking how stupid it is when you had only parked for half an hour too long. Why don't people know that you have had a busy day? The policeman, on the other hand, seems to have nothing better to do with his time than saunter about giving innocent people parking tickets. Policemen, you think, should be chasing criminals.

Is the 'truth' (what is known) about policemen a fixed, measurable and unchanging (context-independent) thing? Or is it the case that we cannot understand 'policemen' until we examine people's experiences of them?

The different approaches to qualitative research

Qualitative research is not just 'one' approach. In fact, there are a number of apparently different approaches or 'methodologies', such as 'phenomenology' and 'grounded theory'. These are 'apparently different approaches' because, in fact, there is not a lot of difference between them. They are introduced here because an awful lot is written about them and because most qualitative research studies are 'pinned' to one of these approaches. Let's be clear about a couple of things.

1. The difference between qualitative research and quantitative research is huge.

2. The difference between the different approaches to qualitative research is so small that such differences are hardly possible to discern.

New words

Ethnography This is a form of qualitative research. Ethnography is derived from anthropology; it focuses on cultural meanings, how the organisation of society is achieved and the meaning that people find in their culture or society.

Phenomenology This is a form of qualitative research. In practice, phenomenology focuses on the interpretation of 'lived experience'.

Grounded theory This is a qualitative approach that focuses on generating theory on social processes by inductive examination of human experience. It is characterised by a close examination of the data, together with reflection on the way it is being coded (constant comparative analysis). In practice, it is a relatively structured form of qualitative research which arguably comes closest to being a 'method'.

People often look to 'ethnography' or 'phenomenology' to try and find a 'method', a particular way of doing qualitative research; however, for the most part they are disappointed. It is important to understand that these different approaches are not 'methods' (ways of doing research). In fact, they more clearly reflect the different groups of people who practise qualitative research and their different academic fields. We do need to know about 'ethnography' and 'phenomenology', etc. because people talk about them all the time and we want to be able to understand what researchers are talking about. Once this is done, we will be able to look at the practical ways in which qualitative research can be carried out.

Qualitative research articles can seem quite easy to understand. However, to really 'understand' qualitative research we need to appreciate how the research was done and why it was done in a particular way. It is at this point that qualitative research begins to look a little complicated. Qualitative researchers usually 'pin' their research to a particular philosophical position on the nature of knowledge. These philosophical positions just 'begin' to point to a 'way' of collecting and analysing data (to a method) – but they only 'begin' to do so; so it is that there is no clearly defined 'method' (way of doing) qualitative research.

One might imagine, then, that there would not be much point in wallowing too deeply in the nuances of phenomenology or ethnography. However, qualitative researchers seem to love nothing better than wallowing in their respective philosophical backgrounds. This contrasts markedly with quantitative research where very little time is spent debating or examining the various methods and where it is usually simply a case of choosing the best method. There is one simple reason for this disparity, and this is that there are no clearly defined qualitative methods. Because of this, it is much more difficult to justify the means chosen to 'do' a particular qualitative study. Qualitative researchers are just trying very hard to make their research look legitimate. In almost perfect contrast, in quantitative research, method and methodology are often used interchangeably, because there is not a lot of theoretical underpinning to the method chosen. Basically, the methodology is just common sense (it's 'logical'). In this way, a randomised control trial is randomised and controlled because this 'works' to control the variables in question and to reduce the effect of any spurious variables.

Qualitative research is stuffed full of theoretical underpinning. Qualitative research in use today rests on a more or less philosophical understanding that developed within anthropology, sociology and philosophy (Astin and Long 2009). This can make it seem quite hard to understand, especially as much of the original philosophical work is now quite old and was written in a deeply philosophical style, and in 'dense' German (McConnell-Henry *et al.* 2009). The philosophers in question were also prepared to invent their own terminology where they felt it necessary, and this further complicates their work. Some qualitative researchers claim that we should adhere rigidly to the qualitative methodologies (the theoretical background) from which modern qualitative research is derived (Frank and Polkinghorne 2010). However, I will attempt here to provide a purposefully pragmatic overview of the core philosophical (methodological) approaches used in qualitative research. I suggest that we take a pragmatic view of this material, for healthcare practitioners are rightly pragmatic and practice-focused people and it follows that their research should be pragmatic too. Smith *et al.* (2011, p. 39) argue that:

> For many years, discussions of the relative merits of generic and theoretical approaches to qualitative research have divided researchers while overshadowing the need to focus on addressing clinical questions

> ... over-adherence to, and deliberations about, the philosophical origins of qualitative methods is undermining the contributions qualitative research could make to evidence-based health care ...

Nevertheless, it is important to understand something of the background to qualitative approaches to research and the core methodological principles to which qualitative research still holds. This is the case, not least because researchers will make reference to this in their writing.

There are three main types of qualitative research: phenomenology, ethnography and grounded theory (Campbell and Roden 2010). Our story begins with a German philosopher called Edmund Husserl (1859-1938) and his one-time student, Martin Heidegger (1888-1976). It was the work of Husserl and Heidegger that first gave rise to phenomenology and, arguably, to the whole area of qualitative research.

Phenomenology

Phenomenology attempts to explain or reveal human experiences. The word 'phenomenology' comes from the Greek 'phainomenon' φαινόμενον (thing or phenomenon) and simply means 'the study of a phenomenon'. In practice, however, phenomenology is the study of the lived experience of a particular thing, or phenomenon.

There are two key approaches within phenomenology: the Husserlian approach and the Heideggerian approach. There are also two key, later developments of phenomenology, namely ethnography and grounded theory.

New words

Positivist paradigm The notion that the world is chiefly an objective and measurable place. Positivism reflects our notion of 'science' as it developed from the Reformation. Quantitative research largely accepts this positivist perspective.

Constructivist (interpretive) paradigm The notion that much of the world is 'open to interpretation', that there is no objective truth or measurable facts, and that instead 'truth' is something that we perceive to be there. In this way, we all see things differently, and what is true for one person may not be true for another. Qualitative research largely accepts this interpretive approach.

Husserl developed phenomenology because he was dissatisfied with the traditional and positivist (quantitative) ways of describing the world. He found that much that was human experience ('lived experience') could not be described or researched using a traditional positivist approach. Husserl rejected the positivist notion that the world only consisted of objective truth (facts). Husserl argued from the perspective of Cartesian duality (René Descartes 1596–1650) that there was a separate mind and body ('duality') and that it was therefore legitimate, even within a positivist paradigm, to study the experience of the mind. In this, Husserl never abandoned a belief that (in a Cartesian sense) at least half the world was factual and objective (McConnell-Henry *et al.* 2009).

Focusing on 'the mind', Husserl developed phenomenology in an attempt to explain or reveal subjective experience. Husserl referred to his work as 'transcendental phenomenology' to indicate that it 'transcended' the traditional view of the world as positivist (subject to quantitative research). Despite Husserl's position that his new phenomenology 'transcended' the traditional positivist view of the world, he remained keen that his new approach be accepted by the scientific fraternity. For this reason he maintained that phenomenological research should be open to objective scrutiny. An important distinction between Husserlian phenomenology and later developments (chiefly those of Martin Heidegger) is that in Husserlian phenomenology the researcher will try to hide his or her own feelings and experience (put them aside or 'bracket' them) to remain objective.

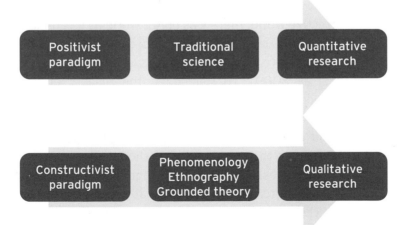

Figure 7.1 The relationship between the perspectives of positivism and constructivism and the two forms of research in use today.

Phenomenology was further developed by Martin Heidegger, who referred to his version of phenomenology as 'hermeneutic', from the Greek 'hermeneuo' (ἑρμηνεύω), meaning 'I interpret' or (in practice) 'understand by interpretation'. This is quite a useful word because it: (1) differentiates Heidegger's ideas from those of Husserl, who maintained an emphasis on there being a degree of objectivity in phenomenological research; and (2) because it reflects the notion that 'truth' as we experience it may not have an objective (measurable) equivalent and that therefore it is legitimate for the researcher to place his or her own 'interpretation' on qualitative data. In Heidegger's version of phenomenology, interpretation is legitimate and there is no pretence of 'objective' analysis of the data. Koch (2006) suggests that researchers should accept and be open about their values and preconceived ideas on the phenomenon being researched and that these values, rather than getting in the way of an objective analysis (which is not in any case the goal), actually make the research meaningful. Koch suggests that (2006, p. 92):

> One of the basic tenets of philosophical hermeneutics is that a dialogue takes place between researcher and participant . . . acknowledging that the researcher . . . brings to the analysis her or his own preconceptions.

However, it is always necessary that the researcher makes explicit the thinking that has led to the interpretation of the data. The reader does not have to share the researcher's perspective or their interpretation, but it should be possible to see how the researcher came to his or her conclusions.

Heidegger rejected the notion of Cartesian duality (a separate mind and body, separate objective and subjective world). Heidegger insisted that there was no such thing as an objective world; there was only a world as it is understand and experienced by people. To Heidegger, the world cannot be measured objectively and there can therefore be no such thing as interpretation-free research (McConnell-Henry *et al.* 2009). To Heidegger, the researcher is an active participant where his or her own experiences are made explicit during the data collection and analysis stages. Consequently, Heidegger rejected the idea that the researcher should 'bracket' (put aside) experience, beliefs and presuppositions, but suggested instead that the researcher should embrace these feelings and take them into the research. Heidegger suggested that the researcher's prejudices, values, beliefs, etc. legitimately exist as an interpretation of reality and are not an obstacle to research. Koch (2006, p. 92) suggests that '*we take value positions with us into the research process. These values, rather than getting in the way of research, make research meaningful . . .*'.

Heidegger's hermeneutic phenomenology has probably had the greatest influence on the development of qualitative approaches, and its influence can be seen in every qualitative study today, even those otherwise labelled as ethnography, grounded theory, etc.). McConnell-Henry *et al.* (2009) make the point that all qualitative researchers seek to explore 'lived experience' and it is this notion, free from the constraints of positivism, that most clearly characterises Heidegger's contribution to the development of qualitative research.

Differences between Husserlian and Heideggerian approaches		
	Husserlian	Heideggerian
Objective/subjective	Phenomenological reduction (bracketing) – researcher tries to be neutral	Hermeneutic cycle – movement back and forth between the data and the analysis, continual process of questioning and examination
Context	Context not important	Context all important
Truth	Aims to expose truth via description	Concerned with interpretation of the human understanding of truth. There are multiple truths, or truth has a 'multiplicity of layers' (Campbell and Roden 2010)
Method	Sees merit in a structured approach with clearly defined methods	No defined method

Research example: phenomenological research in healthcare

Larsson, I., K. Liljedahl *et al.* (2010). 'Physiotherapists' experience of client participation in physiotherapy interventions: a phenomenographic study'. *Advances in Physiotherapy* **12**(4): 217–223.

In this study, Larsson and Liljedahl used a phenomenological study to describe physiotherapists' views on client participation. The study found that physiotherapists had to use three different modes of practice in their interaction with clients; these were collaboration, guidance and expertise.

Ethnography

Ethnography literally means 'people painting'. It developed from the early anthropologists who researched primitive tribes and other communities by living with people and immersing themselves in their culture and traditions (known as 'fieldwork'). Typically, this would involve a lengthy process, collecting data over months and years. Naturally, the anthropologists would analyse their data, often obtained from dialogue of one sort or another, on a continuous basis, as the data was obtained. The combined process of data collection and analysis would be terminated when new data no longer added anything to the analysis, a stage often called 'data saturation'.

Ethnography is related to 'interactionism', a term introduced by Herbert Blumer (1900-1987). Interactionism is an approach to fieldwork which (Gobo 2011):

- focuses on 'meaning' in the context of behaviour;

- takes the actor's (participant's) point of view;

- studies the actor in their own cultural situation;

- focuses on process instead of structures;

- avoids seeing behaviour in term of stereotypes of behaviour, class, race, etc.;

- generalises from descriptions to theory (is inductive).

Ethnography involves being physically immersed in the natural setting of the participants. It usually attempts to build a picture of the language, relationships and social meanings used by a group of people sharing a common cultural identity (such as 'nurses'). As is the case with phenomenology, the researcher may seek to minimise the effect of their own beliefs, etc. (called 'critical ethnography') or may choose not to do so.

Like anthropologists, ethnographers will tend to have an active role in the data collection process (fieldwork). This is typified by their frequent use of 'participant observation', in which the researcher takes on a similar role to that of the participants included in the study. Ethnography has become more popular recently, though perhaps not in healthcare. One can see popular ethnographies produced for television and which involve television presenters living or working with particular groups of people such as accident department staff, fire-fighters, etc. Ethnography is also about 'observation in the natural setting' (Gobo 2011, p. 25). As such, ethnographers tend to avoid using interviews because the actor (participant) is not in their natural setting when they are communicating with the researcher. In this way, techniques that take place outside the natural setting are said not to be ethnographic.

Perhaps the key difference between ethnography and phenomenology is that the former is a very sociological process. Because of this, ethnography is more interested in social groups, culture and society than it is in the individual. Ethnography could be used in healthcare to study the 'culture' of healthcare, for example, but it is certainly less used than are phenomenological and grounded theory approaches. It should not surprise us that healthcare researchers tend to be more interested in individuals than they are in culture. Nevertheless, we come close to ethnography when we ask questions such as 'How do nurses think about (this issue)?' or 'How do limbless soldiers view their disability?'. Here, we may interview nurses or soldiers and obtain individual accounts from them – but we are chiefly interested in building up a picture of 'nurses' or 'soldiers'.

Research example: ethnographic research in healthcare

Thwala, S. B., L. K. Jones *et al.* (2011). 'Swaziland rural maternal care: ethnography of the interface of custom and biomedicine'. *International Journal of Nursing Practice* 17(1): 93–101.

Thwala *et al.* used an ethnographical research study to examine Swazi women's views on western and traditional healthcare models. The study found that, while Swazi women embraced western medicine, they had not given up their use of traditional understanding of illness and treatment in pregnancy.

Grounded theory

Grounded theory was developed by Barney Glaser and Anselm Strauss (Glaser and Strauss 1967). Glaser and Strauss looked at the then implementation of ethnography and phenomenology and created from this a qualitative 'method'; that is, a structured approach to qualitative research. Grounded theory kept the emphasis on inductive research and ethnography's focus on social pro-cesses (rather than individual experience), but did so while including a new 'aim', which was to develop theory. Grounded theory seeks to create theory from interpretation of human experience of a particular phenomenon. This theoretical position can then be used to guide future research, thus providing a mechanism for generalising the results of qualitative research. Strictly, grounded theory, as it was constructed by Glaser and Strauss, is 'sociological' in that it is more concerned with society, culture and the way that people interact than it is about individual human experience. However, grounded theory has been subject to much development and many researchers choose to adopt just a selection of its characteristics in their own work.

In practice, grounded theory has the following characteristics:

- It seeks to develop theory about social processes.

- The literature is reviewed after the analysis has been commenced. This is so that the researcher is not influenced by existing knowledge; this is meant to be compliant with the inductive nature of the research.

- Sampling is determined as the data collection progresses (known as 'theoretical sampling') and ends when there is 'data saturation' (when new data does not add to the developing theory).

- It has stages that are more closely defined than is the case with other qualitative approaches. The analysis of data involves:
  - open coding – to identify 'categories' (broad terms that summarise parts of the data);
  - axial coding – to identify links between the categories;
  - selective coding – to find the core (or main) category into which the other categories link.

- Data collection and theory-building are concurrent, enabling a 'constant comparative analysis' where the researcher moves between the data and the analysis, constantly developing the analysis and re-checking the data to ensure that the analysis reflects the data.

The purpose of grounded theory is to produce theory from data. In practice, however, grounded theory research seldom produces anything close to a 'theory'. It is more usual for the research to produce constructs (ways of viewing things) that can at least loosely be applied to future research and to practice. However, this does not really go beyond what other qualitative research will tend to do. Similarly, while Glaser and Strauss's (Glaser and Strauss 1967) original work did suggest a fairly structured 'method', grounded theory in healthcare research has often been conducted in ways that have allowed ideas from other qualitative approaches to be used. The modern development of grounded theory has seen it more or less merge with other qualitative approaches. Even grounded theory's focus on social interaction and social processes is now hard to discern in the research literature.

However, even this is really not the whole story. In practice, healthcare researchers often use the term 'grounded theory', meaning simply inductive qualitative research. Glaser and Strauss published their work at a time when nursing and the other non-medical healthcare disciplines were developing academically. Glaser and Strauss provided a methodological structure to what had previously only existed as complex philosophical positions, chiefly of Husserl and Heidegger. The freshness of Glaser and Strauss's work, the fact that it was published in English, that it had 'methodological structure' and that therefore it seemed more legitimate to a positivist and developing healthcare profession – all had the effect of making it popular. So, the term 'grounded theory' became popular but the detail of Glaser and Strauss's methodology did not. In practice, there are two interpretations of the term 'grounded theory', a purist one that adheres to the characteristics cited above, and a 'popular' one, where 'grounded theory' is just a general term for inductive qualitative research. If only by accident, Glaser and Strauss's work has popularised and legitimised qualitative research in healthcare. This occurred despite that fact that grounded theory has its sociological position on interpreting culture and society rather than individual human experience. Nevertheless, without this seminal work, qualitative research in healthcare might never have achieved acceptance.

A history lesson

It might come as a surprise even to seasoned academics that qualitative research has existed for millennia. Qualitative research is often assumed not to predate its 'first' proponent, Edmund Husserl, 1859–1938. Most people think that it is quite a new approach. However, we should note that historians have been analysing text for just about as long as people have studied history – that's quite a long time. As far as I am aware, no one ever used statistics to analyse the ancient Egyptian papyri or the Dead Sea Scrolls. These were examined and analysed using historical research methods that are remarkably similar to the qualitative methods used in healthcare research. Historians will sometimes interview (older) people, using a technique known to them as 'oral history'; this too is very similar to the interviewing techniques commonly used in qualitative research. So, qualitative research is not new, but its use in healthcare is new.

Medicine has only existed as a 'scientific' discipline since about the 17th century. A medical text by Thomas Phayre, published in 1540 (Bowers 1999), gives examples of charms and semi-precious stones being used to treat disease. Since the 17th century, medicine mostly concerned itself with 'hard science' and published little about patients' feelings and concerns. For many years, nursing and the other healthcare disciplines took their lead from medicine. However, something happened around the 1970s that would change all that: nursing, and the other non-medical health disciplines, became more 'academic'. University courses began to materialise and were led by practitioners with degrees (mostly) in the social sciences. After all, it was not possible to study at university before the courses had been set up.

A good number of nurse academics in the 1970s had studied sociology. These people became familiar with social philosophy and with notions that challenged the positivist view of the world. In most cases, this material (from which ideas central to qualitative research were derived) got no further than their pencilled lecture notes. However, these budding nurse-sociologists also came across some 'new' work by Glaser and Strauss (1967), called 'grounded theory'. This was refreshingly easy to understand, was written in English and argued that researching people's lived experience was both doable and legitimate. Nurses had always been interested in patients' experiences and much less in their bacteria, anaemia and histology. Here was a new form of research that was exciting in that it could enable nurses to research things in which they were really interested. The fact that these students became Britain's (essentially) first nurse academics, leading new degree courses in nursing, had the effect of 'spreading the word' about qualitative research. Qualitative research in nursing was born and the message spread to other healthcare disciplines as they too brought their training courses into the universities.

From the beginning, nursing viewed qualitative research pragmatically. Nurses were not 'precious' about the philosophical history of grounded theory; they were not concerned with where grounded theory 'had come from' philo-sophically, they were just concerned with what practical use could be made of it. So it is that to the sociologist, grounded theory is a distinct form of qualitative research and one that has to be delineated from other qualitative perspectives. To many healthcare practitioners, grounded theory is 'qualitative research', the new, the refreshed, the legitimate, qualitative research. To healthcare practitioners, it is perfectly possible to claim to be using grounded theory while actually using methods that Glaser and Strauss never described. This can cause much concern among purist sociologists – but there is little evidence that this concern is shared by healthcare academics or practitioners. Ironically, it is the healthcare disciplines that are truly 'inductive', concerned, as they are, with the practical nature of patient and client experience. So it can be argued that, while grounded theory came from deductive-centric sociology, its proper home is with inductive and pragmatic healthcare researchers.

> ### Research example: grounded theory research in healthcare
>
> Livingstone, W., M. Thea *et al.* (2011). 'A path of perpetual resilience: exploring the experience of a diabetes-related amputation through grounded theory'. *Contemporary Nurse: A Journal for the Australian Nursing Profession* **39**(1): 20-30.
>
> Livingstone *et al.* used a grounded theory approach to examine the experience of amputees. The aim was to generate theory that would help practitioners to understand how amputees are likely to experience life after their amputation. The research found that amputees experienced a sense of grief, loss and shock postoperatively but that, despite this, they developed a sense of 'moving forward' in their lives, a sense characterised by hope and endurance.

Mixed and pragmatic methods

Mixed methods can mean the use of a mixture of quantitative and qualitative approaches – sometimes seen in 'triangulation' studies where two or more different methods are used to access the same phenomenon. Mixed methods can be used to adopt some of the positivist principles of quantitative approaches, as in the inclusion of a hypothesis or the use of a deductive approach. Qualitative researchers are not always ignorant of the phenomenon they are researching. Grounded theory in particular aims to produce theory that can then be used to guide future studies in the area. Where this happens, a researcher may well be coming from a theoretical position rather than accepting a position of ignorance of participants' experience.

Mixed or pragmatic approaches are arguably a lot more common than they appear to be. We have seen that researchers often feel the need to justify how they designed their study and how they analysed the data. They do this by making reference to what they argue is the study's philosophical underpinning, usually relating their study to phenomenology, grounded theory or ethnography. Sandelowski (2010) suggests that researchers often claim to use methods from phenomenology, for example, when in fact their study fails to use phenomenological principles or methods. Sandelowski (2010, p. 78) suggests that:

> **Methods are re-invented every time they are used ... there can be no execution of any method that perfectly conforms to any textbook description of it ... indeed, there is no 'it'; there is no bounded entity constituting a pure method.**

Mixed methods may be used within a pragmatic approach. In a pragmatic approach (pragmatic paradigm) the research question is paramount and there is little or no strict adherence to a particular methodology. In this way, a researcher may use ideas in both phenomenology and grounded theory, and even input some positivist ideas at the same time, to develop a methodological approach designed to address the research question. Pragmatists will argue that a method is good if it works. In this way MacInnes (2009, p. 589) suggests that 'what works determines the method'. Smith *et al.* (2011) argue that there has been a preoccupation with philosophical theory in qualitative research and that healthcare researchers should focus their efforts on meeting their study aims, rather than complying with a particular philosophical approach.

In qualitative literature, there is an uneasy relationship between the qualitative purists and those who advocate that mixing up qualitative approaches can be a good thing. It is probably the case that qualitative approaches used within sociology tend to be purist in nature and regard phenomenology and ethnography, etc. as essentially philosophical positions rather than methodologies (McConnell-Henry *et al.* 2009). However, healthcare practitioners tend to be much more open to flexible interpretations of some of the methodological approaches discussed in this chapter. This is, perhaps, not surprising, given the pragmatic nature of their work. Certainly, the pragmatic approach is well legitimised and well used in healthcare research. MacInnes (2009) goes as far as suggesting that the 'pragmatic paradigm' should be considered alongside purer qualitative and quantitative approaches, to create a 'third' approach to research.

Research example: a mixed-methods approach in healthcare research

Smyth, T. and S. Allen (2011). 'Nurses' experiences assessing the spirituality of terminally ill patients in acute clinical practice'. *International Journal of Palliative Nursing* **17**(7): 337–343.

Smyth and Allen used a mixed methods approach that involved the use of a questionnaire and non-structured interviews. The research examined nurses' understanding of patient spirituality. It was found that the nurses did not understand the term 'spirituality'. However, nurses did recognise that patients had needs that were less technical and more 'humane'. In this sense, nurses did practise spiritual care but without recognising it as such.

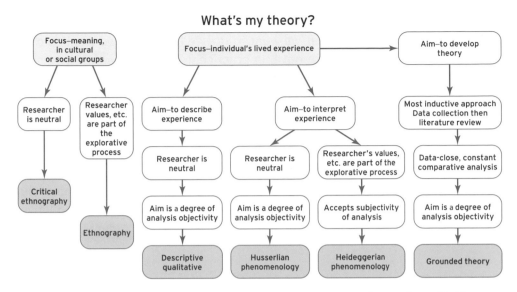

Figure 7.2 The main characteristics of the most commonly used qualitative approaches to research.

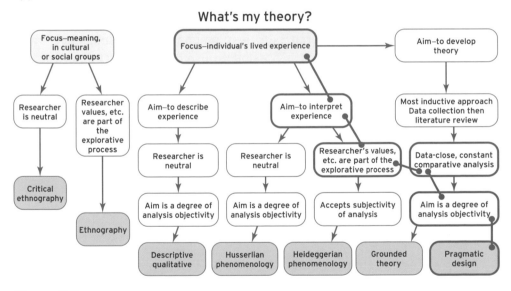

Figure 7.3

Figure 7.3 shows a qualitative design that is close to the principles of Heideggerian philosophy but that adopts the analytical techniques associated with grounded theory. We should bear in mind that healthcare is chiefly an 'inductive' process; it is seldom guided by theory but is orientated toward the practice issues it faces every day. The choice of approach reflected by this chart would seem 'upside down' to many academic disciplines more used to using theory to guide what they do. However, the healthcare practitioner will not be surprised by the 'inductive' (upside down) approach used in this chart. In this situation, we know what we want to do, we know why we want to do it (because it will 'work'), but we have, in practice, to work out what 'theory' is most closely associated with what we have chosen to do. It is worth noting that this is much more difficult than adopting a theory (like grounded theory) and simply doing what that theoretical approach tells us to do (a deductive approach). This difficulty is reflected in the fact that, when writing up their research, healthcare PhD students can often be seen spending much time trying to work out what theory they have used in their research. This is normal, and reflects that fact that healthcare practitioners are pragmatic people who deal in pragmatic things, inductively. Not only is their data collection inductive, but the way they deal with methodology (as in this chart) is inductive too.

Other qualitative approaches

Qualitative descriptive research

Qualitative descriptive research puts less emphasis on a subjective inter-pretation of the data. Indeed, it is possible to use descriptive statistics to, for example, 'count' the number of times the words 'sad' and 'happy' are used in a conversation. Sandelowski (2010) notes that this form of qualitative research is closest to the positivist paradigm and, as such, is purposefully light on theory and deliberately close to the data (little 'interpretation' of it). While acknowledging that some interpretation of the data is necessary, qualitative

> ### Research example: qualitative descriptive research in healthcare
>
> Parvizy, S. and F. Ahmadi (2009). 'A qualitative study on adolescence, health and family'. *Mental Health in Family Medicine* **6**(3): 163–172.
>
> Parvizy and Ahmadi use a descriptive qualitative technique to explore the mental health hazards in adolescent Iranian life. The research involved using purposeful sampling and interviews. It was found that there were three main groups of risk factors: a widening generation gap, effective parenting and the family's financial situation. The study concludes that parents need to com-municate more effectively with their adolescent children and that both parents and adolescents need knowledge about healthy adolescence.

descriptive studies will tend to use thematic or content analysis (more structured forms of analysis). It is certainly worth noting that qualitative research does not have to abandon a positivist perspective and that it is possible to conduct qualitative research in a way that seeks to preserve objectivity.

Discourse analysis

'Discourse' is a pattern of thinking, represented by language and that can be used to explore the social structure of a group of people. Discourse analysis is used in an attempt to understand how language is used to reflect meaning in society and within cultural groups. Nicholls (2009b) suggests that discourse analysis could be used to identify the way that medicine uses 'medical language' to retain power in the interaction with patients. Discourse analysis has no strict definition but is chiefly sociological in context and aims to achieve an understanding of social groups by their use of a common (culturally bound) language. Discourse analysis does not seek to understand or interpret individuals' experience and, perhaps for this reason, is less widely used in healthcare research. However, discourse analysis can be used to look at the ways in which practitioners communicate with clients and patients and the 'language' that is used by patient groups to reflect their common identity.

Research example: discourse analysis in healthcare research

Hayter, M. (2007). 'Nurses' discourse in contraceptive prescribing: an analysis using Foucault's "procedures of exclusion"'. *Journal of Advanced Nursing* **58**(4): 358-367.

Hayter used discourse analysis to study the way in which advice on contraceptives was given to women attending a sexual health clinic. The study found that nurses used medical language to explain the efficacy of contraceptives but used lay language when explaining side effects. This has the effect of minimising the importance of the side effects.

Post-modern/post-structural research

Post-modern/post-structural research takes the view that there is no coherent, structural way of explaining things. Post-modern researchers often choose to study the negative impact of societal structures such as 'law' and 'religion' (Nicholls 2009a). This is, arguably, a further development of the qualitative characteristics, of the lack of a pre-determined method and an acceptance of at least a degree of subjectivity in data analysis. Such studies are unusual in healthcare practice, perhaps because there is a need in healthcare for research to have at least some structure and so be seen as providing material for evidence-based practice.

Research example: post-modern/post-structural research in health and social care

McLeod, A. (2007). 'Whose agenda? Issues of power and relationship when listening to looked-after young people'. *Child & Family Social Work* **12**(3): 278–286.

McLeod studied the 'power play' in the interactions between social workers and looked-after children and found that much of the difficulty in communicating with disaffected children lay in the child resisting the adult's agenda and in them trying to impose their own agenda on the relationship. The research indicates that 'listening' can result in the development of a trusting relationship that could increase the effectiveness of communication with these children.

Concluding remarks

This chapter has presented the theoretical underpinning of qualitative research. We have seen that this underpinning comes from some pretty strange sources. We did not begin our career in healthcare expecting to be studying Heideggerian philosophy. We have seen, however, that much of this material exists to provide a rationale for a subjective stance on research. This argument for subjectivity should be seen in a situation where traditional science has sought for centuries to be objective. Nevertheless, it does seem right to question the positivist view of truth and to try and find truth as it is understood and experienced by individuals. Certainly, there is a place for qualitative research, founded as it is on the notion that people's experience is centrally important and that the world of human beings cannot be understood by looking at the world but only by looking at the human beings who are experiencing that world.

Summary ──────────────────────────────●

- At first glance, qualitative research can seem easy to understand, but just under the surface things become quite complex. This complexity exists largely because 'methods' (how to do qualitative research) have never been properly identified.

- Qualitative research sees the world as it is experienced by individuals. It is not the phenomenon that is important but how that phenomenon is experienced.

- Ideas presented in this chapter see everyone as different and people as too complex and variable to study using traditional scientific methods.

- There are a number of different forms of qualitative research, the most popular being ethnography, phenomenology and grounded theory.

- The differences between ethnography, phenomenology and grounded theory are minor and, in practice, largely unimportant to healthcare researchers. Nevertheless, it is necessary to be familiar with the different approaches discussed in this chapter. This is because the lack of clear method in qualitative research causes researchers to cling somewhat tenaciously to what theoretical material does exist.

- Healthcare researchers often design qualitative studies that take a pragmatic view of the underlying philosophies. In the final analysis, all that matters is that the research 'works'.

Summary of the most common approaches to qualitative research		
Approach	Philosophical underpinning	Practical characteristics
Ethnography	• Roots in anthropology • Aim is to describe and explain social function within a social or cultural group, the experience of belonging to a social group	• Data is collected through immersion (continually being a part of) with the people being studied. Uses 'participant observation'

Phenomenology	• Philosophical roots in Husserlian and Heideggerian philosophy • Aim is to explore the lived experience of individuals and to see the 'truth' as it is experienced by individuals	• Data is collected using mainly interview and focus groups • Data can be analysed by using a structured approach (codes and themes) or by a less structured immersion/crystallisation approach but that always involves interpretation and reflexivity
Grounded theory	• Philosophical roots in ethnography and phenomenology • Focuses on the social processes that occur in human interactions • Aims to develop theory inductively	• Interviews and focus groups often used for data collection • Data is analysed by continuously comparing codes and themes with the data

Further reading

Astin, F. and A. F. Long (2009). 'Qualitative research: an overview'. *British Journal of Cardiac Nursing* **4**(8): 390-393.

Campbell, S. and J. Roden (2010). 'Research approaches for novice nephrology nurse researchers'. *Renal Society of Australasia Journal* **6**(3): 114-120.

Frank, G. and D. Polkinghorne (2010). 'Qualitative research in occupational therapy: from the first to the second generation'. *OTJR: Occupation, Participation & Health* **30**(2): 51-57.

MacInnes, J. (2009). 'Mixed methods studies: a guide to critical appraisal'. *British Journal of Cardiac Nursing* **4**(12): 588-591.

McConnell-Henry, T., Y. Chapman *et al.* (2009). 'Husserl and Heidegger: exploring the disparity'. *International Journal of Nursing Practice* **15**(1): 7-15.

Nicholls, D. (2009). 'Qualitative research: part one - philosophies'. *International Journal of Therapy & Rehabilitation* **16**(10): 526-533.

Nicholls, D. (2009). 'Qualitative research: part two - methodologies . . . second in a three-part series'. *International Journal of Therapy & Rehabilitation* **16**(11): 586-592.

Sandelowski, M. (2010). 'What's in a name? Qualitative description revisited'. *Research in Nursing & Health* **33**(1): 77–84.

Smith, J., H. Bekker *et al.* (2011). 'Theoretical versus pragmatic design in qualitative research'. *Nurse Researcher* **18**(2): 39–51.

Smythe, L. and L. S. Giddings (2007). 'From experience to definition: addressing the question "what is qualitative research?"'. *Nursing Praxis in New Zealand* **23**(1): 37–57.

References

Astin, F. and A. F. Long (2009). 'Qualitative research: an overview'. *British Journal of Cardiac Nursing* **4**(8): 390–393.

Bowers, R. (1999). *Thomas Phaer and The Boke of Chyldren*. London, Arizona State University.

Campbell, S. and J. Roden (2010). 'Research approaches for novice nephrology nurse researchers'. *Renal Society of Australasia Journal* **6**(3): 114–120.

Frank, G. and D. Polkinghorne (2010). 'Qualitative research in occupational therapy: from the first to the second generation'. *OTJR: Occupation, Participation & Health* **30**(2): 51–57.

Glaser, B. G. and A. Strauss (1967). *The Discovery of Grounded Theory: Strategies for Qualitative Research*. Chicago, Aldine.

Gobo, G. (2011). 'Ethnography'. In D. Silverman (ed.) *Qualitative Research*. Los Angeles, Sage.

Hardyment, C. (1995). *Perfect Parents: Baby Care Advice, Past and Present*. Oxford, Oxford University Press.

Hayter, M. (2007). 'Nurses' discourse in contraceptive prescribing: an analysis using Foucault's "procedures of exclusion"'. *Journal of Advanced Nursing* **58**(4): 358–367.

Klopper, H. (2008). 'The qualitative research proposal'. *Curationis* **31**(4): 62–72.

Koch, T. (2006). 'Establishing rigour in qualitative research: the decision trail'. *Journal of Advanced Nursing* **53**(1): 91–100.

Larsson, I., K. Liljedahl *et al.* (2010). 'Physiotherapists' experience of client participation in physiotherapy interventions: a phenomenographic study'. *Advances in Physiotherapy* **12**(4): 217–223.

Livingstone, W., M. Thea *et al.* (2011). 'A path of perpetual resilience: exploring the experience of a diabetes-related amputation through grounded theory'. *Contemporary Nurse: A Journal for the Australian Nursing Profession* **39**(1): 20-30.

MacInnes, J. (2009). 'Mixed methods studies: a guide to critical appraisal'. *British Journal of Cardiac Nursing* **4**(12): 588-591.

McConnell-Henry, T., Y. Chapman *et al.* (2009). 'Husserl and Heidegger: exploring the disparity'. *International Journal of Nursing Practice* **15**(1): 7-15.

McLeod, A. (2007). 'Whose agenda? Issues of power and relationship when listening to looked-after young people'. *Child & Family Social Work* **12**(3): 278-286.

Nicholls, D. (2009a). 'Qualitative research: part one – philosophies'. *International Journal of Therapy & Rehabilitation* **16**(10): 526-533.

Nicholls, D. (2009b). 'Qualitative research: part two – methodologies . . . second in a three-part series'. *International Journal of Therapy & Rehabilitation* **16**(11): 586-592.

Parvizy, S. and F. Ahmadi (2009). 'A qualitative study on adolescence, health and family'. *Mental Health in Family Medicine* **6**(3): 163-172.

Porter, S. (2007). 'Validity, trustworthiness and rigour: reasserting realism in qualitative research'. *Journal of Advanced Nursing* **60**(1): 79-86.

Sandelowski, M. (2010). 'What's in a name? Qualitative description revisited'. *Research in Nursing & Health* **33**(1): 77-84.

Smith, J., H. Bekker *et al.* (2011). 'Theoretical versus pragmatic design in qualitative research'. *Nurse Researcher* **18**(2): 39-51.

Smyth, T. and S. Allen (2011). 'Nurses' experiences assessing the spirituality of terminally ill patients in acute clinical practice'. *International Journal of Palliative Nursing* **17**(7): 337-343.

Thwala, S. B., L. K. Jones *et al.* (2011). 'Swaziland rural maternal care: ethnography of the interface of custom and biomedicine'. *International Journal of Nursing Practice* **17**(1): 93-101.

Watson, J. B. (1928). *Psychological Care of the Infant and Child*. London, Allen and Unwin.

Chapter 8
Qualitative research – how exactly is it done?

CHAPTER OBJECTIVES

The objectives for this chapter are to:

- Provide a simple step-by-step list showing the stages in the qualitative research process

- Outline the characteristics of recruitment (selection), data collection, transcription and analysis

- Discuss ways in which we can judge the trustworthiness of qualitative research

- Provide a simple checklist for use when judging the trustworthiness of qualitative research.

Chapter outline

In the last chapter, we looked at the theoretical underpinning of qualitative research. This chapter will look at how qualitative research is done and how we can begin the review or judge the quality of qualitative research.

Doing qualitative research

One of the first questions that people ask about qualitative research is 'How does one go about doing it?' or 'What are the stages in the qualitative research process?' In practice, however, to undertake qualitative research, we need to be able to work without a concrete list of 'this is how you do it' steps. Campbell and Scott (2011) make the point that there is no 'recipe' for qualitative research. There are two points worth noting:

- It is hard to 'plan' qualitative research because the research is inductive, so we cannot anticipate what the data will look like. Because we don't know what the data will look like, we cannot fully anticipate how we will analyse the data.

- Unlike quantitative research, qualitative research does not possess a universally accepted and coherent methodology.

Klopper (2008) suggests that any qualitative study is designed by conducting it and that qualitative design has 'an emergent nature' (p. 63). In addition, we have already noted (in Chapter 7) that many healthcare researchers adopt a 'pragmatic' approach to method and therefore do not stick rigidly to any methodological roots that may exist. In this way, they may happily 'mix' ideas from grounded theory, phenomenology and ethnography. This 'mixing' of methods is especially common in healthcare research, perhaps because healthcare researchers tend not to come from a purist background and as a result are not 'precious' about theory. Indeed, Nicholls (2009, p. 586) suggests that 'It is theoretically possible to imagine that we might devise as many methodological approaches as there are researchers.'

This mixing of methodological approaches occurs despite some authors' (Frank and Polkinghorne 2010) call for researchers to adhere more closely to the philosophical roots of their chosen approach rather than to develop their own methodological stance. On the other hand, some would argue that to allude to 'a way of doing' qualitative research is to disdain the very nature of it. The trouble is, this eclectic or even *laissez-faire* stance makes it almost impossible to discern 'how to do' qualitative research simply by looking at existing studies.

Yet, somehow, we need to move from this to a position where we can at least know how to begin to 'do' qualitative research. You can see opposite a simple 'to do' list. You may be surprised at how simple it is and how much it seems 'just common sense'. However, this should not surprise us, for all good research is simple and all good research is, indeed, just common (logical) sense.

Qualitative researcher's 'to do' list

1. Identify the research question, e.g. 'How do people with a deformity experience the healthcare system?'

2. Try to answer the following questions, but don't worry if the answers only come to you as you conduct your research.

    - Are you interested in individual experience or how groups of people interpret social systems, society or culture?

    - Are you trying to describe human experience or are you trying to interpret it?

    - Are you trying to develop a theory or are you content to describe or interpret the experience of your participants?

    - Do you want your ideas and values to be 'hidden away' and for you as researcher to be as objective as possible, or do you want to be open about your ideas, values and experiences and to use these attributes in communicating with your participants?

    The answers to these questions will help you to relate your study to a particular named approach to qualitative research (discussed in the previous chapter) or to an eclectic mix of more than one approach.

3. Do a literature review – even if you want to use an inductive approach, there is still no point in being purposefully ignorant of the existing literature. Find out whether your subject has been researched before and, if so, how it has been researched. *Note*: the purist grounded theory researcher will want to leave the literature review until the data analysis commences.

4. Decide how best to address your research question. If you are interested in lived experience you will probably choose to interview people who have had the experience in question. However, you should also consider focus groups, diaries, observation, etc.

5. Decide how you can best recruit participants to the study.

6. Decide on a broad approach to analysis. This largely rests on how structured you want the analysis to be.

7. Consider ethical implications of what you wish to do.

8. Discuss your research plans with others, make appropriate modifications and seek ethical approval.

9. Begin collecting the data.

10. Transcribe the data as it comes in.

11. Look at your data as it 'comes in' rather than when you have collected it all.

12. Conduct an 'initial reading' of the text, followed by a closer scrutiny.

13. Identify anything in the text that is interesting, seems 'key', typical, different, odd, etc.

14. Label (code, categorise) the above. Try to use labels that summarise the text somehow, but bear in mind that these labels will evolve and change as you re-examine the text and look at more text as it comes in. Note that some labels will be descriptive while others will be conceptual.

15. Grounded theory researchers will at this stage search the literature for existing theory (theoretical sensitivity); this may give new insight and cause further analysis to be needed.

16. Look for 'negative cases', data that seem to disagree with the developed codes, categories or themes. Ensure that these are fully explored.

17. Keep a journal (log, diary). Record every single thought, decision and change of label – what you thought, what you did, why you did it.

18. Regularly review your labels (categories, themes), re-examine text you have already labelled and review the labelling.

19. Identify labels that can be grouped together to form higher-level labels.

20. Identify what association or patterns may exist between labels and groups of labels.

21. Identify broad categories of labels that effectively and accurately reflect the data (proto-theories). It is these that will exist as the summary of the analysis and that will be communicated to others when the research is published.

22. Lastly, this is a cognitive exercise, so always 'think'. Never let the 'process' or the 'task' take control. Always think: What is this, what is going on here, are my labels (codes, categories) really reflecting the text, are there any patterns here? Always question 'Am I getting this right?'

The above is a simple and logical list. You did not need to understand Heideggerian phenomenology (etc.) to be able to follow this list and perhaps put it into action. However, we need some understanding of theoretical underpinning to be able to make choices in method and to be able to communicate the research to others.

The following sections will look at key stages in the qualitative research process:

- Recruitment (sampling)

- Data collection

- Analysis.

Recruitment (sampling)

Qualitative research is interested in the lived experience of individuals. We have seen that qualitative research sees everyone and everyone's experiences as unique and conditional upon the contexts of time and space (our experience is not a static thing). In practice, this means that there is no 'population' that we want to sample. We are not looking for a small number of participants who will represent a large number of people. Most qualitative researchers are happy to argue that their research has been the study of (for example) 10 participants. There is no need for a nice big number of participants; indeed, qualitative studies can be 'biographical' and have only one participant. However, although qualitative studies do not 'sample' a population, the word 'sample' is in such common use that researchers will sometimes use it. Normally, however, the word 'recruitment' is used. So, participants are 'recruited' to a study.

Participants are recruited using a wide variety of means. It is not uncommon for qualitative researchers to research people with whom they are familiar. A ward sister, interested in patients' experience of oncology diseases, might already know the participants whom she recruits to the study. It is possible to advertise, asking, for example, for people who were ambulance drivers in the war to come forward to share their experiences. Another technique is called 'snowballing' (Mansour 2011), where one participant contacts others known to him or her and asks them if they will consider being part of the study.

Magilvy and Thomas (2009) point out that participants in qualitative studies must meet the following criteria:

- *have experienced* the phenomenon under examination;

- be *able* to communicate their experiences to the researcher;

- be *willing* to communicate their experiences.

It can certainly be difficult to locate suitable participants and to find people who will agree to talk about issues that are important to them. It can also be difficult to retain participants in a study, especially if it is a more longitudinal study. While there is no need for the 'sample' to be representative of a population of similar people, researchers usually want to be able to argue that the conclusions to their study have relevance to other studies and to practice generally. Nevertheless, there are few of the sampling issues found in quantitative studies. We do not need to worry about a biased sample, we do not need to estimate what size of sample we will need and we certainly don't need a 'large' sample to convince others of the worth of our study.

Data saturation

Prior to the data collection stage, qualitative researchers cannot usually determine what number of participants will be required. Instead, the researcher will carry on collecting data from new participants until a point is reached where no new material is being added to the analysis. This is called the data saturation point and it signals the completion of the data collection.

Data collection in qualitative research

This section looks at the most commonly used data collection methods, namely:

- in-depth interviews;
- focus groups;
- qualitative diaries;
- observation.

In-depth interviews

The interview is a key approach within qualitative research. It is especially useful in providing rich data that can successfully reflect the lived experience of the participant. The interview is useful where we do not know much about the participant's experience and where we are chiefly interested in exploring the participant's own version of things – the participant's lived experience. It is not surprising that the interview has been the benchmark and cornerstone of qualitative research.

Conducting a good interview takes practice and experience. It can be hard to keep the participant appropriately focused. There is a skill in achieving this. If this focus is not achieved, one can easily spend 2 hours or more talking about nothing much at all. Additionally, the process of 'prompting' the participant for further or deeper information is an important one if the researcher is not to be left with nothing more than a collection of 'Yes', 'No' responses.

Interviews can be emotionally exhausting, both for the participant and the researcher. Qualitative research often deals with emotionally challenging material and it is not uncommon for participants to find themselves revealing thoughts that they had never considered deeply before. In this way, the interview has the potential to be damaging, and interviews are often distressing. There needs to be time allowed for silences and pauses, allowing the participant to reflect, perhaps for the very first time, on his or her experiences. Pauses are also useful to provide a brief but essential 'rest' from the proceedings. Interviews may be distressing for the researcher too. It is not uncommon for qualitative researchers to be investigating matters that are close to their own heart. Smythe and Giddings (2007) state that:

> You come up against yourself in qualitative research. The studies have an impact on you (p. 41) . . . Qualitative research is risk taking because you face-up to 'you' in practice. You face-up to the patients as well, not as the person with liver cancer but as Joe, not as the Parkinsonian patient, but as Mary . . . (p. 43).

Interviewers need the following skills (Banner 2010; Bulpitt and Martin 2010):

- ability to communicate clearly
- adequate knowledge of the focus area (need to be able to understand what the participant is communicating and be able to share an understanding with the participant)
- ability to listen to the participant actively
- ability to clarify and probe sensitively
- empathy with the participant – the researcher needs to feel what the participant is feeling
- ability to be reflexive; that is, for the researcher to 'know themselves' and where they stand on the issues central to the research.

Anyone who researches an emotionally sensitive subject (and health researchers often do) needs to have 'come to terms' with the emotionality of that subject before they start researching it with others. A researcher needs not only to be able to 'deal with' emotive material; they also need to be 'able to deal with other people dealing with it'. Reflexivity also helps to reduce researcher bias by making the researcher aware of his or her own values, etc.

However, all this is not easy, and the developing nature of qualitative research can make it hard for the participant and the researcher to fully 'know' what emotional challenges may be just around the corner.

The type of questioning used in an interview can be structured (unusual), semi-structured or non-structured. Examples are:

- structured – 'How long have you worked in intensive care?'

- semi-structured – 'How do you feel when a patient gets better and is able to go home?'

- unstructured – 'Tell me about your time as a nurse.'

In practice, interviews often contain a mix of question types. Nevertheless, researchers like to cite the main style of their interviews using one of the above classifications. Qualitative research seldom uses a fully structured interview. Most qualitative interviews in healthcare research use a mixture of semi-structured and unstructured questions. More structure is used when we know what questions we want to ask; less structure is used when we accept that we don't know much about the participant's experiences and so we don't know what questions to ask – we are only familiar with the 'area' we want to explore. Wholly unstructured interviews are like 'guided conversations' (Whiting 2008). Usually, interviews have some structure, where prompts are used to ensure that rich data is collected. Prompts can look like this:

Interviewer (prompt): Tell me about your time as a nurse.

Interviewee: I worked from the mid-1950s, having trained at St Paul's hospital. I remember my first job was on an orthopaedic ward. I recall being terrified on my first day (laugh).

Interviewer (probe): Tell me about your first day.

It is important to avoid using leading questions like 'Were you nervous on your first day because you lacked confidence?' Leading questions have two main problems: they reflect the researcher's ideas, not the participant's ideas, and they can 'throw' the participant, causing him or her to focus on what is believed to be the researcher's interest and to think that their own experiences are not valued.

Whiting (2008, p. 38) discusses the use of different types of probes:

- Silence – allows the participant to think

- Echo – the researcher repeats what the participant has said to encourage elaboration

- Verbal agreement – as in, 'Yes, I understand, go on.'

- Tell me more – the interviewer directly asks the participant to tell more

- Leading – asks a question that leads in a particular direction

- Baiting – gives impression of being aware of something the participant is referring to – tends to encourage further discourse on the matter.

The most common approach taken by qualitative researchers is to have an interview plan containing prompts rather than questions. The prompts serve to keep the interview focused rather than to seek answers to particular questions. It is important both to stay focused toward the research question and to elicit data that reflects the interviewee's experiences in a reasonably full (or rich) manner. In pursuance of this, the interviewer may well have to review his or her list of prompts both within an interview and for subsequent interviews. This is often needed when it becomes apparent that the interviewees have a key experience not originally anticipated by the researcher. Interviewers need to be both focused and flexible and to have the skills to see where the dialogue is going, to perceive the nuances of conversation that might be hiding a key experience and to probe carefully, sometimes incisively, while always with care for the interviewee's welfare. It takes experience to be a good interviewer; it is certainly not a case of simply asking people questions.

To be in a position of talking with people about their key experience is a great privilege. It is necessary to respect the participant, their experiences and the information that is communicated. In any case, for people to be really open about their experiences, they will need to trust the researcher and a rapport will need to have been established. The environment will need to be both safe and physically and emotionally comfortable.

The interview has four key stages.

1. The interviewer and participant get to know each other. Any questions asked at this stage are non-threatening and non-emotive. The interview format is introduced, with the researcher explaining:

   a. the purpose of the interview;

   b. the anticipated length of the interview;

   c. how confidentiality will be managed;

   d. permission to record the interview;

   e. assurance that it is okay to refuse to answer questions (and that the participant can ask questions).

2. More in-depth questions can be asked. The interviewer is listening and learning all the time. During this stage, a sense of trusted sharing develops.

3. The interview becomes more 'comfortable'. Both parties feel they know each other, they feel they can say things to each other without causing upset or offence. Mutual trust exists. This can be a time for clarifying points and for prompting in directions that may be more sensitive. If the interview goes well, there will be a sharing of interest, just as two people who shared the same experience might communicate together. The interviewee may guide and teach the interviewer.

4. The interviewer begins to close the interview, allowing it to come to an end over a period of time. Here, simpler, non-emotive questions are often re-introduced, as a way of carefully pulling away from the emotive aspects of the discourse. Closing the interview can be difficult for the participant, especially if it is to be the last interview. It is an unusual experience to be able to talk about an important life event and to someone who actually wants to listen. This can be quite therapeutic, and individuals can come to feel that they do not want the interview(s) to end.

Interviews – practical issues

Practical considerations include:

- *The location of the interview*: the interview needs to be somewhere that will allow the participant to relax. This may be in the participant's own home, in their workplace or somewhere else. Often, the participant is encouraged to choose the location. However, the researcher needs to be aware that participants sometimes get upset during an interview and that, because of this, it is sometimes better for the interview to be in a neutral place, like a room at the university. There may also be distractions at home, from the postman calling at the door to children constantly demanding attention.

- *How the interview will be recorded*: researchers usually want to record the interview, not least because the recording allows them to examine the interview over and over again. Video recording has the advantage that it will show the non-verbal communications. Often, a lot can be gained from being able to see the participant's facial expressions. However, participants are often reluctant to be recorded and they will at least need to know that the recording will be kept safe and confidential. Sometimes, the participant will ask for the recorder to be turned off in the middle of the interview.

- *Transcription*: the recording will need to be transcribed (written down). This is very time-consuming. A 1-hour interview will take the average researcher at least a day to transcribe.

- *English quality and transcribing*: the quality of spoken English is seldom as good as written English. There is a tendency to 'convert' the transcript into good English and to remove local dialectical words and phrases. However, it is probably better to keep these in the transcript. In fact, much of the original richness of the data is lost when it is written down on paper, and it can be better to do the analysis with both the transcript and the recording at hand.

Interviews – ethical issues

One might suppose that most qualitative research would be risk-free. We are used to thinking of research ethics being mostly concerned with new drugs and interventions that have the capacity to cause bodily harm. It is true that no one was ever killed by being interviewed. However, qualitative enquiry can be damaging. This is partly because of the emergent and unpredictable nature of qualitative research – we never really know where the research will take us, and so it is more difficult to plan for and anticipate difficulties (Houghton *et al.* 2010). Qualitative research often seeks to examine experiences that are deeply personal and traumatic. So, too, it is often the case that participants find themselves in the research interview talking about things they have never discussed before, even with themselves. It is not at all unusual for participants to become upset during the interview. This raises the issue about how participants can be supported and who should do the supporting. Certainly, qualitative research has ethical issues that need careful consideration whenever a qualitative study is planned, and while it is in progress.

Confidentiality is a particular issue in qualitative research. This is because the participant's data is in audible or textual form and is very 'accessible'; someone coming across the data would immediately understand it. The data tends to be sensitive, relating to matters that are deeply personal. It is often the case that researcher and groups of participants already know each other and will continue to know each other after the research is complete. Aspects of interview data may well relate to other participants. Participants may tell the researcher something that raises professional issues. Sometimes, research can deliberately focus on professional issues – a research study into 'healthcare workers' experience of unsafe practice', for example. Situations like this need to be managed very carefully.

There is often a power relationship between the researcher and the participant. Interviews can be used, wrongly, to coerce participants to talk about things they do not really want to discuss. Bulpitt and Martin (2010, p. 14) refer to the 'seductiveness' of the qualitative interview. Here, the opportunity to talk to someone who is ready and eager to listen and to understand, an opportunity often much valued by the participant, 'seduces' him or her into saying things that would not normally have been said. Participants may want to retract and remove from the record something they have said. It may seem a simple thing to do this (and it should be done) and, yet, what the participant wants to retract may be important data for the researcher. The relationship between the researcher and the participant is a fluid one and the researcher needs to be aware of how it is developing.

Example from the literature

Houghton, C. E., D. Casey *et al.* (2010). 'Ethical challenges in qualitative research: examples from practice'. *Nurse Researcher* **18**(1): 15–25.

Houghton *et al.* (2010) show how they dealt with ethical issues that arose during interviews with nursing students. The paper deals with a number of ethical issues that arose. The researchers found that their role as researcher and their role as nurse educator became confused. This caused difficulties with the power relationship and with confidentiality. The authors show how they managed to resolve these issues as the study progressed.

The interview can also be therapeutic for the participant; just talking about something to someone who wants to listen can be a significant experience (Jack 2010). However, this close association between research and therapy is something that researchers in other fields try to avoid, arguing that we need to be clear about whether we are performing the role of researcher or practi-tioner (Bulpitt and Martin 2010). Such clarity is sometimes hard to achieve in qualitative research, but it is important that the researcher constantly bears these issues in mind as the research develops. This requires a continual process of reflection.

The research interview can be a significant experience in its own right. It can expose the researcher to the participant's positive and negative emotions, their dreams and their nightmares. The interview is an immensely useful tool but it should be handled carefully. Training in research interviewing technique can be invaluable. Within the research process, the ability to de-brief and to access peer review and mentorship are useful, perhaps even necessary. This is so, not just for the starting researcher but also for the experienced researcher. Qualitative research takes us to places to which we did not imagine going and which are new to us. This is as it should be and it indicates the value of interviews.

Example from the literature

Bulpitt, H. and P. J. Martin (2010). 'Who am I and what am I doing? Becoming a qualitative research interviewer'. *Nurse Researcher* **17**(3): 7-16.

In this article, Bulpitt and Martin reflect on the experience of conducting research interviews.

Focus groups

Focus groups as a technique evolved in the 1940s, at which time they were mostly used for market research (DiCicco-Bloom and Crabtree 2006). A focus group is a group of individuals, essentially interviewed together. However, the focus group is not a short-cut to doing lots of interviews at once; indeed, of interest here is the way that the group interacts and the material that can be elicited from the discussion between members of the group. In this way, a focus group approach can sometimes elicit material that would not be easy to obtain during a one-to-one interview.

To facilitate discussion, members of the focus group can be encouraged to ask each other questions or to tell the group about their experiences. The role of the researcher is not so much to ask questions but to keep the group's discussion focused and to manage whatever group dynamics may arise. It is not uncommon to have one person who wants to talk all the time and another who doesn't want to talk at all; situations like this need careful management. Rothwell (2010) suggests that a good focus group leader (sometimes called a 'moderator') attempts to lead the group but with minimal involvement and yet in a way that will lead to maximum interaction from the group members.

Recording a focus group and transcribing the content can be a real challenge. An audio recording will not make it clear who is speaking. A video recording, on the other hand, will show who is speaking and it will also show the non-verbal communications and group dynamics (that is, 'how' the group is interacting). However, focus group members often do not like being video-recorded and the video equipment can inhibit dialogue. People are often conscious of 'how they look' on video, even though this may be of no interest to the research. Video needs to be done well if it is to be of any use and, in practice, this can be quite a challenge.

It takes some experience to manage a focus group well and people new to the task should ensure that they have support available to them. The key benefit of focus groups is that they enable interaction between participants and in a situation that is potentially less affected by the power relationship than in a one-to-one interview.

Example from the literature

Bench, S. D., T. Day et al. (2011). 'Involving users in the development of effective critical care discharge information: a focus group study'. *American Journal of Critical Care* **20**(6): 443-452.

Bench et al. describe the use of focus groups of patients and family members to provide insight into issues relating to discharge from critical care to general care and the role that information-giving has on this.

Diaries

Qualitative researchers have always been prepared to consider written material as a useful source of data. Historians, anthropologists and ethnographers have all accepted the use of written material as legitimate. However, to most researchers, it seems natural to study 'lived experience' by communicating with people at interview. Nevertheless, diary and other written material can be useful, especially where:

- participants may be reluctant to be interviewed;
- data need to be collected over a span of time (longitudinally);
- it is needed to augment interview data.

Consider, for example, a researcher wanting to collect data from children aged about 12 years. In an interview situation, it would be difficult to get away from a power differential between the adult researcher and the child participant. On the other hand, when 12-year-old children write a diary, they are on their own and are able to write what they want. Nicoll (2010) makes the point that interviews require the participant to recall experiences and, although the main body of those experiences are likely to remembered, the detail of them is often lost. Diaries, however, can be maintained 'as things happen' and in this way can be more accurate. Diaries can contact both factual information and reflections on events.

Diaries can contain 'prompts' by having different sections, labelled, for example:

- when it happened;

- what happened;

- what you thought about it.

Diaries don't just have to be written on paper. These days diaries often take the form of computer 'blogs'. This use of electronic diaries is well understood, especially by teenagers and young adults.

Diaries can be used alongside interviews; the interview can even be designed to probe aspects of the written diary. The interview(s) can also act to provide encouragement for the participant to continue writing the diary. Dialogue about the diary will have the effect of assuring the participant of the diary's value.

Example from the literature

Holtslander, L. and W. Duggleby (2008). 'An inner struggle for hope: insights from the diaries of bereaved family caregivers'. *International Journal of Palliative Nursing* **14**(10): 478-484.

Holtslander and Duggleby describe the use of diaries with bereaved women. The diaries provided a useful insight into the participants' struggle to find 'hope' in their lives.

Observation

People new to research often start out thinking that observation would be a good way to study people. We need to be clear that there is a big difference between a 'time and motion' study; measuring how many times practitioners wash their hands, and studies that try to understand human experience. Direct observation can take the form of either participant or non-participant observation. Ethnographers and anthropologists may wish to share the time and space of the participants as a key way to understanding the social processes in which they are involved. However, this has not been a popular approach to studying healthcare situations. Here are some of the reasons for this:

- Qualitative research is more interested in experience than it is in human behaviour.

- Most participant and non-participant research has quantitative goals (counting hand-washing).

- Direct observation presents a number of ethical and healthcare organisation political difficulties in relation to patient privacy, etc.

- It is very difficult to obtain on-going consent from anyone who might end up being 'watched'.

Example from the literature

McKnight, M. (2006). 'The information seeking of on-duty critical care nurses: evidence from participant observation and in-context interviews'. *Journal of the Medical Library Association* **94**(2): 145–151.

McKnight used participant observation to study the ways that nurses obtain information. It was found that nurses spent much of their time collecting information about their patients, but they had little time to collect information that they could use to increase their own knowledge or to develop practice.

It can be seen that there are a number of ways in which qualitative data can be collected. In practice, the interview is by far the most commonly used technique. Each technique requires both careful planning and at least a degree of experience. Lastly, it is important that the data collection process does not harm anyone and that we understand that the potential for harm is present. It can be seen that the data collection methods available to us are capable of providing much richer data than can usually be collected using quantitative techniques. Qualitative research has been significantly effective in providing insight into the lives of patients, family members and practitioners. There can be no doubt at all that these methods are effective.

Transcribing the data

While it is not strictly necessary, interview and other oral data are likely to be converted into written text. This is because it is easier to analyse text and it is quite difficult to analyse an audio or video recording directly. Occasionally, interview data are not recorded at all; instead, notes are made during the course of the interview. However, this is unusual and almost always the data collection is recorded and then transcribed into text.

It is important that the transcript is accurate and reflects what was actually said and not what the transcriber thought the participant 'meant' to say. It can be difficult to transcribe language that is often regional and is almost always grammatically imperfect. Sentences that make perfect sense when they are spoken sometimes make very little sense when they are written down. People often make much use of non-verbal language and this is not recorded at all in an audio recording.

Transcribing interviews always takes a considerable period of time. Unfortunately, it is not usually a good idea to give the job to a typist which, in any case, would be very expensive. It is better for the researcher to transcribe the recording and for that to happen shortly after the interview itself.

Analysis in qualitative research

Those new to qualitative research often have difficulty in working out just how they are supposed to analyse textual or interview material. It would be fair to say that looking at published research papers is unlikely to clarify much, for qualitative researchers are often pretty vague about the exact mechanism they employed to analyse their data. There will often be a reference to grounded theory, phenomenology, ethnography or some such thing, but what that means exactly is seldom made clear. Such references are often included to make the work look legitimate, the researcher competent and the analysis robust. We should take glib references to grounded theory, phenomenology, etc. with some scepticism for, if the researcher used an analysis that was methodologically clear and transparent, then they could have communicated that to the reader. All too often, the researcher simply fails to communicate the method used to analyse the data. In such situations, it is fair to surmise that the analysis has been as clear to the researcher as it is to the reader.

We can be sure of one thing; qualitative analysis takes a very long time (Jirwe 2011). It is not at all uncommon for a PhD student to take 6 months to a year to analyse their qualitative data, while those with quantitative data have sometimes completed their statistical analysis in just a few days.

Data analysis in qualitative studies takes one of three broad approaches:

- descriptive or quasi-statistical;

- structured analysis (the use of frameworks, matrices, content analysis, thematic analysis, grounded theory);

- interpretive immersion in the data.

The most common approach in healthcare research is to use some kind of structure, as in thematic analysis. Here, themes are discerned from the data. The researcher then takes the themes back to the data to check their usefulness in summarising and interpreting the data. As new data is read and re-read, the themes are allowed to evolve until a definite set of themes is identified. Sometimes pre-existing codes are used but these are always allowed to develop as the analysis proceeds. The codes are then grouped into categories or themes to develop high level concepts that reflect the data.

Structured approaches (all inductive) include:

- framework analysis;

- thematic analysis;

- interpretive phenomenological analysis;

- grounded theory analysis (characterised by its focus on theory development).

Using some kind of structure enables a degree of objectivity and allows the research to be auditable, opening it to scrutiny. There is no real difference between the structured methods listed above. While they are often described separately, as separate entities, the methods each uses are very similar, even arguably and in practice, the same (see Analysis in practice, below). 'Content analysis' is a convenient term that means 'any form of qualitative analysis' (Twycross and Shields 2008). This seems to be a good and useful overarching term, especially as the differences between one method and other are at best 'minor' and are, arguably, 'indefinable'. In practice, each qualitative analysis is different and that 'difference' is greater than the difference between the items in the above list of methods. It is perhaps because an author will cite 'thematic analysis' as the form of analysis used in his or her study that we think we need to know about 'thematic analysis' and, indeed, that it must exist as a discernible entity. When a lot of researchers say they used thematic analysis, we become sure that thematic analysis must be something real and discernible. However, we would be wrong. What in practice is going on here is that each researcher feels the need to legitimise his or her research by referring it to the literature, and so they use what Rapley (2011, p. 273) calls a 'tag':

> Above all, whatever you read, you realise that it is *de rigueur* to have some kind of tag. You need the right kind of label in your methods section, ideally, one that positions you as competent, so that your work can be nicely categorized.

So, we don't need to worry about what is thematic analysis and what is framework analysis. For they are no more different than a computer monitor and a computer screen, a laugh and a giggle, a street and a road.

A less structured approach (immersion/crystallisation/iterative approach) can avoid using themes or codes at all. Instead, the researcher repeatedly immerses himself or herself in the data in a series of reflective cycles until an intuitive interpretation of the data emerges (DiCicco-Bloom and Crabtree 2006). The complete avoidance of any coding structure is unusual in healthcare research. It can be difficult for the researcher to explain fully how their interpretation of the data can be seen in the data itself.

Software is available to help with qualitative data analysis. However, while just about every quantitative researcher will use statistical software, many qualitative researchers will choose to do their analysis by hand. Qualitative researchers may tend not to enjoy technology much or, as Banner and Albarran (2009, p. 25) politely put it, 'may sometimes suffer from technological conservatism'. Certainly, the benefits of software for qualitative researchers are less clear than is the case for statistical analysis. Software does allow data to be kept all in one place and for several researchers to work on them at the same time. Large amounts of data can be coded and coding structures can be changed on the fly without having to recode everything manually.

Software in use today includes:

Ethnograph, used for coding data: **http://www.qualisresearch.com/**

Nvivo and Atlas.ti, used for both coding data and theory building: **http://www. qsrinternational.com/products_nvivo.aspx; http://www.atlasti.com/**

It might be useful here to consider again the following data analysis 'to-do' list.

Analysis in practice (any paradigm)

1. Look at your data as it 'comes in', rather than when you have collected it all.

2. Conduct an 'initial reading' of the text, followed by a closer scrutiny.

3. Identify anything in the text that is interesting, seems 'key', typical, different, odd, etc.

4. Label (code, categorise) the above. Try to use labels that summarise the text somehow but bear in mind that these labels will evolve and change as you re-look at the text and look at more text. Note that some labels will be descriptive while others will be conceptual.

5. Grounded theory researchers will at this stage search the literature for existing theory (theoretical sensitivity); this may give new insight and cause further analysis to be needed.

6. Look for 'negative cases', data that seem to disagree with the developed codes, categories or themes. Ensure that these are fully explored.

7. Keep a journal (log, diary). Record every single thought, decision and change of label. What you thought, what you did, why you did it.

8. Regularly review your labels, re-read text you have already labelled and review the labelling.

9. Identify labels that can be grouped together to form higher-level labels.

10. Identify what association or patterns may exist between labels and groups of labels.

11. Identify broad categories of labels that effectively and accurately reflect the data (proto-theories). It is these that will exist at the summary of the analysis and that will be communicated to others when the research is published.

12. Lastly, this is a cognitive exercise, so always 'think'. Never let the 'process' or the 'task' take control. Always think: What is this, what is going on here, are my labels (codes, categories) really reflecting the text, are there any patterns here? Always question 'Am I getting this right?'

We should not be anxious about 'doing it right'. There isn't a 'right way' of doing qualitative analysis, there is only the way that best suits the research study in question and that will address the questions that the study aims to answer.

Whatever form of analysis is used, there is an ever-present danger that the participants' accounts will be interpreted in terms of the researcher's own values to the point where the participants would not recognise the interpretation. It should always be possible to 'see' the data within the interpretation provided by the researcher. However, this does not help the reader of qualitative research papers because neither the data nor the lengthy analysis will be there. This does tend to mean that we have to accept the researcher's interpretation of the data. A full 'audit' of the research would in any case be very time-consuming. There is ongoing debate about this issue, with some arguing that the 'art' and subjectivity of qualitative research should be embraced (Rolfe 2006) and others demanding that the analysis should be transparent and auditable (Porter 2007). In practice, researchers need to be able to make it clear how exactly the analysis was performed. Even where that analysis is heavily 'interpreted' it should be possible for the researcher to explain what mechanisms were made to enable the interpretation.

How exactly do I evaluate qualitative research?

Trustworthiness is a qualitative term that means the overall quality of research. Curtin and Fossey (2007, p. 88) define trustworthiness as 'the extent to which the findings (of the research project) are an authentic reflection of the personal or lived experience of the phenomenon under investigation'.

We can examine the quality of quantitative research in relation to internal and external validity and reliability:

- Internal validity (truth; have we correctly measured the thing we set out to measure?)

- External validity (is the study generalisable?)

- Reliability (if we did the study again, would we get the same results?).

However, these terms do not relate well to qualitative research. Qualitative research tends to accept the participants' accounts as inherently valid, seeks not to be generalisable because people are seen to be individuals and it is almost nonsense to think of replicating a qualitative study (reliability) because each study is different (Ryan-Nicholls and Will 2009).

Qualitative studies are very large things that do not lend themselves to publica-tion in academic journals. The effect of this is that such a limited amount of material is presented in a typical article that it is quite impossible to use it to judge the quality of the research. A quantitative study can be communicated succinctly to a journal audience but this is not the case with qualitative studies. There is currently no effective means by which we can judge the quality of qualitative research except through audit. This is not something the reader of journals can do, for an audit must have the whole research project, data, researcher's log, etc. available for scrutiny. So, don't be surprised if you find it difficult to judge qualitative research as it is published in journals properly, for we all do. There is just not enough information there for us to make a judgement. Clearly, this is a problem, for we want qualitative research to be used in relation to 'evidenced-based practice' and for that we need it to be capable of being judged (Porter 2007; Ryan-Nicholls and Will 2009). Perhaps the answer lies in a system of audit where qualitative studies in their entirety can be scrutinised by an expert panel. However, we are some way off finding a solution to this problem and for the time being we have to work with what we have got.

Well-understood things are easy to communicate. Poorly understood things are difficult to communicate. Freud's theory of the subconscious mind and the 'big bang' theory are both quite difficult to understand because no one really understands them. We do not understand either the subconscious mind or how intelligent, experiencing life could be the result of an explosion in space. In the same way, there is a great deal of confusion about qualitative research and how the quality of it should be assessed (Porter 2007; Ryan-Nicholls and Will 2009). It is not complicated because it is complicated but because, like the subconscious mind and the big-bang theory, it is not well understood. This lack of understanding has generated a plethora of descriptive terms, with people making up new terms when they find that existing ones are not useful. For the time being, we will have to live with this. If you find this material confusing, be assured that you are doing very well indeed with it, for you are absolutely right, it is confusing.

Validity (truth)

We have already seen that 'truth' (internal validity) is not seen to exist in positivist terms but only as it is experienced by a person in one time and place. Qualitative studies largely regard material acquired at interview to be inherently true. To the qualitative researcher, internal 'validity' is, instead, seen as the degree to which the interpretation of the data can be seen in the data itself. However, we have already seen that this interpretation can be quite subjective, with this subjective interpretation viewed as being perfectly legitimate. Before

we become too despondent, we should note that 'truth' is pretty hard to measure in any kind of study. Quantitative studies will tend to accept that 'truth'
exists when the variable is measured in the same way on two occasions. In this
way, a questionnaire can include some questions that are repeated. If the participant is being truthful (and not just ticking boxes randomly) they will answer
the repeated questions in the same way. However, consistency does not equal
truth. One can imagine a defendant at a police station consistently telling the
police he did not commit a crime. The police question him again a week later
and he denies the crime again. Does this mean that our defendant is telling the
truth and is innocent? Perhaps not. So, truth in research is a pretty elusive
commodity. Truth is a very slippery phenomenon and we should not fool
ourselves into thinking that it can be identified in any study, however it is done.
In fact, qualitative studies have some advantage over quantitative studies, for
the former tend to claim only that they are interpreting what the participants
choose to tell the researcher. What *is* true is that the participant told the
researcher the things that the participant told the researcher. These things are
recorded and transcribed and we know at least *what* we are measuring.
Conversely, quantitative studies are often less than sure of what it is they have
measured. Consider, for example, the use of a simple pain scale, used to record
a patient's perceived level of pain. Let us say that we have a score of '5'. Two
questions now present themselves: (1) what exactly does '5' pain mean (does
our measurement of pain actually make any sense, even to us); and (2) how
sure are we that we are not measuring 'anxiety' instead, or a mixture of pain
and anxiety? In an important sense, qualitative research does at least get
its information from the 'horse's mouth'; our data is first-hand data, not a
measure of a measure of a measure. Additionally, we do at least know how the
participant has interpreted their experience or at least how they have chosen
to report that experience to us, using their own language and without having
to convert their experience to a number.

External validity (generalisability, transferability)

Qualitative studies do not seek to generalise their results (external validity)
because they are chiefly concerned with the experience of (usually) a small
number of people. To the die-hard qualitative researcher, each person is
unique and is not like other people, or, indeed, even like him or herself across
time and space (our understanding of our experience changes over time). This
causes Barusch *et al.* (2011) to argue that generalisability is the very antithesis
of qualitative research. However, the results of qualitative research can give us
insight into others' experience. Indeed, grounded theory (Glaser and Strauss
1967) fully embraces this argument and makes theory construction its very

aim. On balance, we can see that qualitative research is designed to give us insight into the participant's lived experience. This insight can be useful when we turn to look at other individuals. What qualitative research achieves is a new 'insight' into people who are, for example, physiotherapy patients, parents on a children's ward or people who have had a stroke.

Lastly, qualitative studies do not seek to be reliable. Indeed, it is largely accepted that even if the same data were to be analysed by two different researchers, it would be legitimate for them to come to two different conclusions.

Some have attempted to adapt the terms used above, so that we have, for example (see table):

Measures of trustworthiness (research quality)	
Qualitative term	**Meaning**
Credibility	Similar to 'internal validity'. The degree to which the researcher's interpretation of the data can be justified in the data itself
Transferability	Similar to 'external validity'. The degree to which the concepts, constructs or theory generated by the analysis can be applied elsewhere
Dependability	Similar to 'reliability'. If the study was repeated, similar results would be obtained
Plausibility	The degree to which the researcher's interpretation of the data is likely to be realistic given our existing knowledge
Confirmability	Sometimes used in ethnography. The degree to which it is possible to assess whether the findings flow from the data. (Is the study 'auditable'?)

In qualitative research, there is no sense of 'doing it properly'. Barusch *et al.* (2011, p. 12) suggest that '. . . there is no consensus on what strategies or how many should be used to develop strong qualitative research', and that art exists not only in doing qualitative research but also in judging its quality. This is the case because, in qualitative research, there is no coherent system of methods (Rolfe 2006). It is the case that every qualitative research study is different. However, rigour in qualitative research is said to exist when the reader is able to audit the data collection and analysis. In other words, it should be possible to see exactly how the researcher conducted the research and how they interpreted the data. This interpretation is essentially subjective; however, it should still be possible for the researcher to explain how and why their interpretation was made.

Despite the difficulty in measuring the quality of qualitative research, there are a number of ways in which researchers try to enhance the trustworthiness (overall quality) of their studies. These are summarised in the list below:

- Analysis triangulation

- External audits

- Member checking

- Method triangulation

- Negative case analysis

- Peer debriefing

- Peer review

- Prolonged engagement/persistent observation

- Reflexivity (openness about researcher biases).

Triangulation

Triangulation is the use of more than one method. The term comes from a technique used by surveyors to identify one point in space by relating it to two or more other points whose position is known. Triangulation in qualitative research simply means using more than one technique, either to collect data (method triangulation) or to analyse data (analysis triangulation). Triangulation can be achieved by collecting data from different sources. For example, data could be collected from paediatric staff and from parents of children. Their accounts will be different but it should be possible for the two accounts to be related in a way that makes human sense to us. We could seek to collect data from the parents, at interview, using a qualitative approach but, in addition, we might be able to use a questionnaire to ask questions related to the focus of the research. Again, the data will be different but it might be possible to relate the two sets of data in a meaningful way. This would help to give us confidence in both sets of data. We might choose to collect data both from interviews with participants and also by direct observation of them or perhaps by asking participants to keep a diary of the experiences. I think we can see that method triangulation can work to give us confidence in the data.

Qualitative research usually uses only one method of analysis (probably because it takes such a long time to do) but it might be possible to undertake an analysis that uses a structure of codes and themes alongside one that is more iterative, where text is read over and over again and an attempt is made to summarise it in full text. This latter could be carried out on just a 'sample' of the full text available to the researcher. Again, the results will be different but we would expect to see a degree of commonality or agreement between the results of both analyses and this would tend to give us confidence in the analysis by achieving what Barusch *et al.* (2011) called 'consensus' or 'corroboration'.

External audits

Qualitative research should leave behind it an 'audit trail', which allows others to look at each step of the research in detail and judge its quality. However, the world of research has very few mechanisms for achieving these audits, at least outside PhD programmes. The Cochrane Foundation is looking at ways of achieving this but for the present time qualitative research is only 'HD ready' – good research leaves an audit trail but there is no one currently present to do the audit.

Member checking (participant data validation)

This is not about counting fingers and toes; rather, it is a process whereby one or more aspects of the data or the analysis are shared with the participants to obtain their views on it. At its simplest level, each participant can be given the transcribed interview for them to check that it accurately reflects what was said at the interview. This can be an opportunity for them to add new material or to comment further on things that were said. Often, a summary of the interview or the preliminary results of the analysis of the interview data are given to the participants for their comments. This technique rests on the assumption that results of the analysis should be reflective of the participant's experience as it is understood by the participant. Some take issue with this assumption, arguing that the analysis of the data is a skilled task that only seasoned academics are able to do (Rolfe 2006) and that their analysis can legitimately differ from that of the participant. However, most healthcare researchers are keen to understand how the patient/client sees things and they don't have much time for defining participants' experiences within some clever theoretical paradigm, so we should not be too worried by these concerns.

Negative case analysis

Researchers often get quite excited when they are able to see a pattern of find-ings in their data; that is, they begin to see what is 'really going on' in what is being reported in the data. However, it is at this time that other patterns, which do not agree with the main one, sometimes become apparent. It can be easy to ignore or not give sufficient weight to these 'negative case', parts of the data that do not agree with the researcher's emerging conclusion. Negative case analysis is a deliberate attempt to focus on those aspects of the data that do *not* comply with other ideas arising from the text. In this way, negative case analysis can be seen as 'thoroughness' in the analytical process.

Peer debriefing and peer review

Peer debriefing is a process similar to peer review, commonly used in profes-sional practice. It can involve the researcher reporting the planned research or the research-in-progress to one or more other individuals who are not directly involved in the study. This enables the research to be considered with 'fresh eyes' and for difficulties and researcher biases to be made explicit and examined. Peer review is a similar term but often indicates a more formal process.

Prolonged engagement with participants/persistent observation

It is a characteristic of qualitative research that the researcher will spend a lot of time with participants. This is particularly true of ethnography, where data is collected from participants in their natural environment. In any qualitative study, the data collection takes a long time. This is generally seen to be a good thing, for the more time one spends with participants, the richer will be the data and the more the researcher will tend to understand the data as the participants understand it.

Reflexivity

Jootun *et al.* (2009, p. 42) calls reflexivity 'one of the great pillars of qualitative research'. While in quantitative research most of the 'thinking' goes into the planning stage, in qualitative research that thinking is present from the beginning to the end of the study. Reflexivity is characterised by constantly asking oneself the questions 'What do I know?' (of the data) and 'How do I know it?' (what interpretive process is going on here?). Jootun *et al.* (2009) make the point that, while qualitative research and analysis are essentially subjective in character, the mapping of the reflexive process can at least make the research open and transparent.

Reflexivity is similar to the notion of 'reflective practice', often used by healthcare practitioners to question their own practice and their interpretation of it and to construe ways of improving it. In almost exactly the same way, a qualitative researcher will continuously question the approach they are using and their interpretation of the data. The researcher will keep a record of this reflective activity and so should be able to report a summary of it. Such a summary can tell the reader how the researcher's ideas on the data developed over time. This helps to make the research process transparent. Peer debriefing can be used here to ensure that the reflective process is open to change, even while it is developing.

In addition, the following research characteristics should also be present:

● Analysis method described

● Audit trail

● Data collection method described

● Ethical issues discussed

● Evidence that data saturation was reached

● Recruitment (sampling) rationale provided

● Thick description achieved (see below).

(Some would also add that the research is referenced (tagged) to a particular theoretical approach (i.e. to phenomenology or grounded theory).

Thick description

Thick description is a detailed account of the data and analysis. Often researchers will use quotes from the data to illustrate how the summary of their analysis can be related back to the original data. Curtin and Fossey (2007) suggest that thick description is evidenced by:

● a detailed description of the context of the study;

● a rationale for the chosen method;

● full documentation of the data collection;

● a detailed description of the analysis.

Here is an excerpt from the qualitative analysis of data from Fernandez and Wilson's (2008) study on Maori mothers' smoking habits. The researchers identified themes that were common to the interview data. Here, we offer an example of the theme 'being a mother'. In this way, being a mother is suggested as one factor that influenced the Maori women to stop smoking.

> Motherhood had special significance for participants. Being a mother was particularly significant during their experiences of pregnancy, and in response to positive feelings about their children. Their babies' health was consequently identified as being important. Therefore, quitting or not smoking during pregnancy was perceived as maternal acts of protecting and nurturing their unborn babies. Some participants acknowledged their gratitude to their babies for 'making' them quit:
>
> 'I always give up when I'm pregnant' (Participant A).
>
> 'I thank my baby; she made me give up smoking' (Participant B).
>
> Participants also agreed that, apart from their own health, their children were the most important reason for them to stay smoke-free:
>
> 'Health has kept me motivated [to stay smoke-free] and my kids' (Participant E).
>
> Fernandez and Wilson (2008, p. 32)

Audit trail

Qualitative research is essentially a subjective process. However, the subjectivity of the process means that it needs to be open to scrutiny. For this reason, qualitative researchers log every 'step and turn' of the research. This will include a description of the cognitive steps the researcher took while interpreting the data. Such an audit trail helps to make the study open, transparent and auditable by others.

When we judge the quality of a qualitative study, we ask two main questions (Koch 2006).

1. Are the researcher's conclusions firmly grounded in the data (can we relate the conclusions to the data)?

2. Are the conclusions explained by the researcher's interpretive scheme (do they make sense, bearing in mind the researcher's explanation of their interpretive strategy)?

It remains the case that qualitative research, with its lack of clear methods, can appear sloppy (Ryan-Nicholls and Will 2009). Healthcare practitioners are used to seeking clear 'evidence' to support their practice. Qualitative research, with its emphasis on subjective interpretation of human experience, can seem to fall short of 'evidence'. However, Wiart and Burwash (2007) maintain that qualitative research can provide clinically relevant information about patient values and experiences. They suggest that (p. 215): 'In the reality of clinical practice, knowing why patients choose not to participate in an intervention is as important as knowing about its efficacy.'

How to review qualitative research – a checklist

Now we know what qualitative researchers 'do' when they conduct their research. We also know what we can expect to be present in a study in relation to its 'trustworthiness'. The resulting checklist can help us to make a judgement on the quality or trustworthiness of qualitative research.

A	Thick description (clarity)	Comments	YES	NO
A-1	Does the study have a clear focus and goal, is the research problem clearly stated?	It is important, even with qualitative research, that the research has a clear focus. However, the focus may well be in the form of 'Find out how individuals in a group of epilepsy sufferers experience healthcare intervention'		
A-2	Is there evidence that the research has considered the existing literature, either at the beginning of the study or at some point in the course of the study, to ensure that the study 'builds on' existing knowledge?	Qualitative research is almost always strongly inductive. As such, it often tries not to be influenced by existing ideas, constructs and theories that may be present in the literature. However, it is still always necessary to build on and add to existing knowledge, and the existing literature should therefore be used at some point in the study.		

A	Thick description (clarity)	Comments	YES	NO
A-3	Is the method of recruitment clearly identified?	The study should make it clear how participants were selected, what were the inclusion and exclusion criteria. While the 'sample' need not be strictly representative of any 'population', there is usually a desire to be able to apply the findings to other people, situations or future studies.		
A-4	Are ethical issues clearly identified?	Were support mechanisms in place in situations where participants might experience emotional distress?		
A-5	Is the data collection procedure (e.g. interviews) described clearly? Is it clear what was done and is there a clear rationale provided for what was done?	Both the process and the rationale should be clear and should be compliant with the research question.		
A-6	Is there evidence that data saturation was reached?	This is the point at which new data is not adding anything to the analysis. Data collection should not stop before data saturation is reached.		
A-7	Method – general: is there reference to a method or philosophical underpinning?	The research may refer to ethnography, phenomenology grounded theory, etc. or to an eclectic mix of methods, but the method should always be clear.		
A-8	Method – focus: does the research make it clear whether the focus is on individual lived experience or to group, culture or societal function?	There is a fundamental difference between trying to interpret lived experience (as in phenomenology) and trying to examine or interpret the meaning in social groups (defining the social group by the meaning individuals have in it), as in ethnography.		

A	Thick description (clarity)	Comments	YES	NO
A-9	Method – bracketing: is it clear whether the researcher tried to be neutral (bracketing) or to be open about values and other attributes?	We need to be clear about whether the researcher tried to be neutral (as in unbiased) or whether s/he openly accepted his or her values, experience, assumptions, etc. and used these (purposely) to influence the research.		
A-10	Has the researcher used one or more of these? ● Analysis triangulation ● External audits ● Member checking ● Method triangulation ● Negative case analysis ● Peer debriefing ● Peer review ● Prolonged engagement/ persistent observation ● Reflexivity (openness about researcher biases)	At least one should have been used. There should also be a rationale for their use or for not using each or most of the procedures in the list.		
A-11	Has the researcher left an audit trail?	The researcher should have kept a log of each stage in the research process and each stage in the interpretation (cognitive) of the data.		
A-12	Analysis method: is the exact method of analysis detailed?	It should be possible to be clear about how exactly the data were analysed. For example, were codes, themes or categories developed from the data?		

B	Summary measures of trustworthiness		1-5*
B-1	Credibility	Similar to 'internal validity'; the degree to which the researcher's interpretation of the data can be justified in the data itself.	
B-2	Transferability	Similar to 'external validity'; the degree to which the concepts, constructs or theory generated by the analysis can be applied elsewhere.	
B-3	Dependability	Similar to 'reliability'; if the study was repeated, similar results would be obtained.	
B-4	Plausibility	The degree to which the researcher's interpretation of the data is likely to be realistic given our existing knowledge.	
B-5	Confirmability	Is the study 'auditable'?	

* It may be useful to provide a numeric score to each item in this last part of the table. This will provide us with a meaningful summary measure. Some will regard this as being 'beyond the qualitative pale', but if it is useful, then we should do it.

Concluding remarks

This chapter has cut through some of the very confusing terminology used to describe qualitative research. The list at the beginning of the chapter on 'how to do qualitative research' really does indicate that it is actually quite easy to do and to understand. You now understand qualitative research pretty well. However, out there in the intellectual wilderness there is still a lot of confusion and a notable lack of clear, universally accepted qualitative methods. There really are about as many ways to do qualitative research as there are published qualitative research papers.

We should bear in mind that quantitative methods have been developing at least since the 17th century and that qualitative methods are still comparatively new. We have already noted that qualitative approaches in healthcare are really not much older than Glaser and Strauss's publication of grounded theory (Glaser and Strauss 1967). Grounded theory provoked much excitement at the time and we are still within that first exciting period. This is a time when qualitative research in healthcare is still new and still developing. It is a confusing time because so much is happening; qualitative research in healthcare has barely had time to stand still since the late 1960s. It is, however, a time of enormous opportunity. Eventually, we will have at our disposal both properly validated qualitative research methods and a better understanding of patients and practitioners.

Healthcare professionals are often interested in their patients' feelings and experiences. Our greater understanding of how both illness and intervention are experienced by patients and clients will surely help us to provide better care.

Summary

This chapter has looked at how qualitative research is done and how we are able to judge the quality of completed research. In looking at how research is done, we have seen that qualitative research requires a degree of 'people' skill. Such skill is needed, for example, when we interview people about things that are key experiences for them. Researchers need the skill to keep the interview focused and to probe the participant for the deeper information that qualitative research always seeks. However, we also need to achieve empathy so that we have some insight into what the interview is doing to the participant. We need to be caring and careful and to know when to pull back, to pause the interview or stop it altogether. Such skills are not easily found in the general population but are found amongst healthcare professionals. It has already been suggested that the inductive nature of qualitative research suits the pragmatic healthcare professional well. So, we should not be surprised that qualitative research has blossomed to the degree that it has begun to marginalise traditional scientific approaches to healthcare research.

Further reading

Banner, D. J. (2010). 'Qualitative interviewing: preparation for practice'. *Canadian Journal of Cardiovascular Nursing* **20**(3): 27-30.

Barusch, A., C. Gringeri *et al.* (2011). 'Rigor in qualitative social work research: a review of strategies used in published articles'. *Social Work Research* **35**(1): 11-19.

Curtin, M. and E. Fossey (2007). 'Appraising the trustworthiness of qualitative studies: guidelines for occupational therapists'. *Australian Occupational Therapy Journal* **54**(2): 88-94.

DiCicco-Bloom, B. and B. F. Crabtree (2006). 'The qualitative research interview'. *Medical Education* **40**(4): 314-321.

Houghton, C. E., D. Casey *et al.* (2010). 'Ethical challenges in qualitative research: examples from practice'. *Nurse Researcher* **18**(1): 15-25.

Koch, T. (2006). 'Establishing rigour in qualitative research: the decision trail'. *Journal of Advanced Nursing* **53**(1): 91-100.

McBrien, B. (2008). 'Evidence-based care: enhancing the rigour of a qualitative study'. *British Journal of Nursing (BJN)* **17**(20): 1286-1289.

McConnell-Henry, T., A. James *et al.* (2009). 'Researching with people you know: issues in interviewing.' *Contemporary Nurse: A Journal for the Australian Nursing Profession* **34**(1): 2-9.

Nicholl, H. (2010). 'Diaries as a method of data collection in research'. *Paediatric Nursing* **22**(7): 16-20.

Nicholls, D. (2009). 'Qualitative research: part three - methods.' *International Journal of Therapy & Rehabilitation* **16**(12): 638-647.

Rapley, T. (2011). 'Some pragmatics of data analysis'. In D. Silverman (ed.) *Qualitative Research*. Los Angeles, Sage.

Rothwell, E. (2010). 'Analyzing focus group data: content and interaction'. *Journal for Specialists in Pediatric Nursing* **15**(2): 176-180.

Ryan-Nicholls, K. D. and C. I. Will (2009). 'Rigour in qualitative research: mechanisms for control'. *Nurse Researcher* **16**(3): 70-85.

Smith, J. and J. Firth (2011). 'Qualitative data analysis: the framework approach'. *Nurse Researcher* **18**(2): 52-62.

References

Banner, D. J. (2010). 'Qualitative interviewing: preparation for practice'. *Canadian Journal of Cardiovascular Nursing* **20**(3): 27–30.

Banner, D. J. and J. W. Albarran (2009). 'Computer-assisted qualitative data analysis software: a review'. *Canadian Journal of Cardiovascular Nursing* **19**(3): 24–27.

Barusch, A., C. Gringeri *et al.* (2011). 'Rigor in qualitative social work research: a review of strategies used in published articles'. *Social Work Research* **35**(1): 11–19.

Bench, S. D., T. Day *et al.* (2011). 'Involving users in the development of effective critical care discharge information: a focus group study'. *American Journal of Critical Care* **20**(6): 443–452.

Bulpitt, H. and P. J. Martin (2010). 'Who am I and what am I doing? Becoming a qualitative research interviewer'. *Nurse Researcher* **17**(3): 7–16.

Campbell, S. and J. Scott (2011). 'Process of conducting qualitative research'. *Nurse Researcher* **18**(2): 4–6.

Curtin, M. and E. Fossey (2007). 'Appraising the trustworthiness of qualitative studies: guidelines for occupational therapists'. *Australian Occupational Therapy Journal* **54**(2): 88–94.

DiCicco-Bloom, B. and B. F. Crabtree (2006). 'The qualitative research interview'. *Medical Education* **40**(4): 314–321.

Fernandez, C. and D. Wilson (2008). 'Maori women's views on smoking cessation initiatives'. *Nursing Praxis in New Zealand* **24**(2): 27–40.

Frank, G. and D. Polkinghorne (2010). 'Qualitative research in occupational therapy: from the first to the second generation'. *OTJR: Occupation, Participation & Health* **30**(2): 51–57.

Glaser, B. G. and A. Strauss (1967). *The Dscovery of Grounded Theory: Strategies for Qualitative Research*. Chicago, Aldine.

Holtslander, L. and W. Duggleby (2008). 'An inner struggle for hope: insights from the diaries of bereaved family caregivers'. *International Journal of Palliative Nursing* **14**(10): 478–484.

Houghton, C. E., D. Casey *et al.* (2010). 'Ethical challenges in qualitative research: examples from practice'. *Nurse Researcher* **18**(1): 15–25.

Jack, B. (2010). 'Giving them a voice: the value of qualitative research'. *Nurse Researcher* **17**(3): 4-6.

Jirwe, M. (2011). 'Analysing qualitative data'. *Nurse Researcher* **18**(3): 4-5.

Jootun, D., G. McGhee *et al.* (2009). 'Reflexivity: promoting rigour in qualitative research'. *Nursing Standard* **23**(23): 42-46.

Klopper, H. (2008). 'The qualitative research proposal'. *Curationis* **31**(4): 62-72.

Koch, T. (2006). 'Establishing rigour in qualitative research: the decision trail'. *Journal of Advanced Nursing* **53**(1): 91-100.

Magilvy, J. K. and E. Thomas (2009). 'Scientific inquiry. A first qualitative project: qualitative descriptive design for novice researchers'. *Journal for Specialists in Pediatric Nursing* **14**(4): 298-300.

Mansour, M. (2011). 'Methodological and ethical challenges in investigating the safety of medication administration'. *Nurse Researcher* **18**(4): 28-32.

McKnight, M. (2006). 'The information seeking of on-duty critical care nurses: evidence from participant observation and in-context interviews'. *Journal of the Medical Library Association* **94**(2): 145-151.

Nicholl, H. (2010). 'Diaries as a method of data collection in research'. *Paediatric Nursing* **22**(7): 16-20.

Nicholls, D. (2009). 'Qualitative research: part two - methodologies . . . second in a three-part series'. *International Journal of Therapy & Rehabilitation* **16**(11): 586-592.

Porter, S. (2007). 'Validity, trustworthiness and rigour: reasserting realism in qualitative research'. *Journal of Advanced Nursing* **60**(1): 79-86.

Rapley, T. (2011). 'Some pragmatics of data analysis'. In D. Silverman (ed.) *Qualitative Research*. Los Angeles, Sage.

Rolfe, G. (2006). 'Validity, trustworthiness and rigour: quality and the idea of qualitative research'. *Journal of Advanced Nursing* **53**(3): 304-310.

Rothwell, E. (2010). 'Analyzing focus group data: content and interaction'. *Journal for Specialists in Pediatric Nursing* **15**(2): 176-180.

Ryan-Nicholls, K. D. and C. I. Will (2009). 'Rigour in qualitative research: mechanisms for control'. *Nurse Researcher* **16**(3): 70-85.

Smythe, L. and L. S. Giddings (2007). 'From experience to definition: addressing the question "what is qualitative research?"'. *Nursing Praxis in New Zealand* **23**(1): 37-57.

Twycross, A. and L. Shields (2008). 'Research update. Content analysis'. *Paediatric Nursing* **20**(6): 38.

Whiting, L. S. (2008). 'Semi-structured interviews: guidance for novice researchers'. *Nursing Standard* **22**(23): 35-40.

Wiart, L. and S. Burwash (2007). 'Qualitative research is evidence, too'. *Australian Journal of Physiotherapy* **53**(4): 215-216.

Chapter 9
How to succeed with your essay on research and evidence-based practice

Most university healthcare programmes contain a module on evidence-based practice or research. This book was written because many students find research difficult to understand. The real test of that understanding is the essay that many students have to write on the subject. Of course, such modules and courses vary in what they demand of students. However, many students find themselves having to review one or more research papers or to examine the evidence that supports an aspect of practice. Students should always seek advice first of all from their own module tutors. However, this chapter contains some general advice on how to write a competent essay.

The assessment is set because the professions recognise the importance of research and want you to be able to understand research and to use it in your practice. However, there are one or two difficulties that are inherent in an assessment of this kind. First, your faculty staff would probably prefer you to get some experience in real-life research. This is not usually possible because it would take too long, there isn't enough research going on to provide the experience and cohorts of students are often too large. It is because of this that your faculty may decide to ask you to review a piece of research or to look at the degree to which an aspect of practice is supported by evidence. This seems reasonable enough, until one realises that students are being asked to critique or evaluate something of which they have no experience. In this respect, it is like being asked to tell someone how to drive a car when you have never sat in one yourself.

So, it is not that research is complex or difficult to understand. The issue here is that you have probably never been involved in any research. However, the healthcare disciplines are developing and are not yet perfect; while they are still imperfect, there will be challenges to face.

Unfortunately, what we have discussed so far is not the only issue. These assessments are not only difficult to write; they are also difficult to mark. There are two broad ways in which an examiner can regard your essay:

- How well your essay works as an essay

- How well you have understood the research.

In the second of the two categories, there may be an expectation that emphasises the research design and methodology or one that emphasises the analysis. In any case, what is expected of you should be identified very clearly in your module or course handbook. If you are still unclear about what is expected of you, ask someone. It can also be useful to get together with other students who are keen to do well with this assessment, meet several times and work things out together.

Tips on writing a good essay on research and evidence-based practice

Some students enjoy studying and others prefer to pick up their knowledge as they go along. Students on placement, however, are rather unlikely to become involved in research and so research is something that benefits from a reasonable amount of reading. The more you read about research, the more you will become familiar with the language of research. You will then be able to use this language in your essay and it will be clear to the examiner that you are familiar with and comfortable with the language of research. This is time-consuming and needs to be built into your busy schedule. This is one essay that should not be left to the last moment.

> Read about research. This is time-consuming and needs to be built into your busy schedule. This is one essay that should not be left to the last moment.

Just as you should try to become familiar with the language of research, it helps a lot if you can become familiar with the clinical issue that you will discuss. So, for example, you may want to write your essay about the research on post-operative pain. In this case, make sure you know about postoperative pain. After all, you will want to introduce the subject of postoperative pain in your essay and your conclusion will be about postoperative pain. A lot of your essay will actually be about postoperative pain, so become familiar with it as a subject. This will also help you to under-stand the research. If you are able to,

> Become familiar with the clinical issue that you will discuss.

you can save yourself a lot of time by choosing to look at the research available on an aspect of practice with which you are already familiar.

Try to be up to date with your general essay-writing skills. This is no time to have to struggle with that as well. If this isn't possible, make sure that at least

> Make sure that you reference properly.

you reference properly. Get a copy of your faculty's referencing guidelines, read those guidelines and stick to them. Good referencing is often considered to be more important in the field of research, and the examiner may expect this to be reflected in your essay.

It may be that you have written all of your previous essays without obtaining any tutorial help. You may be nervous about asking a tutor to critique your work. However, this is one essay on which help is decidedly useful. Go and see your tutor as soon as possible, at the beginning of the module, find out what help he or she is able to offer and then use that help. Your tutor will guide

> Go and see your tutor as soon as possible, find out what help he or she is able to offer and then use that help.

you about what you need to include in your essay and will help to explain some of those research terms. Be brave: see your tutor and ask for feedback on your essay. Use whatever resources your faculty makes available to you.

Understand that your research critique is an exercise in communication, just like every other essay you have written. Your essay should tell a story and have a beginning, a middle and an end. Your essay should be about something and have a clearly transparent purpose. It can be useful to ask yourself what you are trying to communicate and why.

> Your essay should be about something and have a clearly transparent purpose.

Your essay should be in three parts:

1. An introduction (discussion)

2. A review of the research (description)

3. A discussion of the implications of the research (analysis).

> Your essay should be in three parts: an introduction, a review, a discussion.

In the introduction, consider including two pieces of discussion. The first should be about the need and purpose of research in healthcare. The second should introduce the clinical problem (the focus of the research, such as post-operative pain).

If you are reviewing research, make sure that you include some discussion on:

> Make sure that you include some discussion on the need for the research, the design and methodology and what the research found.

- the need for the research and the background to it;

- the design and methodology of the research – that is, how it was done;

- what the research found: don't shy away from the statistical analysis – it is important that you are able to say what the research actually found.

You may have been asked to select a piece of research on which to base your essay. You may think it best to go to a relatively easy-to-understand journal, but this may not be such a good idea. You may not be confident in differentiating a good study from a poor one. Instead, get your study from an aca-

> Get your study from an academic journal.

demic journal; at least then you can be reasonably sure that the research will be of good quality. Knowing that a study is likely to be of good quality will help enormously when it comes to critiquing it. Should your chosen study have used regression analysis? If your chosen study came from a reputable academic journal, then it is very unlikely that the researchers will have chosen an inappropriate analysis. You can be reasonably sure that the regression analysis was the right thing to do. Now all you need to do is to look up regression analysis to get a definition of it that you can understand.

By now, you will be used to critiquing things. Your faculty staff have encouraged you to question everything and to avoid being descriptive. However, you should question and critique only mate-rial that you understand. Imagine that someone took you into theatre and you were able to watch a world-renowned

> Question and critique only material that you understand.

neurosurgeon operate on someone's brain. After the operation was over, they took you to one side and said, 'Now, how well do you think they did that operation and what could they have done better?' Doubtless you would think that an odd question. So it is with research, except that your assignment may actually ask you to evaluate a piece of research. This is one occasion when it may be safer to stick to description. There is a danger that, in critiquing the research, you may simply succeed in exposing your own lack of knowledge. It is probably the case that the research has been carried out appropriately and that the researchers themselves have identified what weaknesses and limitations there may be in the research. Remember that in any good journal, the research paper will have been peer-reviewed by at least one person and probably two people with research and academic experience. So, be careful about critiquing the study and be prepared to be a little more descriptive than you are with your other essays. You can balance this descriptiveness by putting argument and analysis into the discussion section of your essay. The discussion section will be where you look at the implications of the research for healthcare, for patients and for future research. Here you can relate the research and its findings to practice, and question and critique as much as you wish.

It may be that you find a research study that seems not to be perfect and you are confident that you understand it well enough to provide a critique. Even here, you should pause and consider whether the problems with the research were because of the researchers' error. It is often the case that a more perfect or more robust design and method would be fine in theory but impossible to conduct in practice. Healthcare research often deals with human participants who will not readily fit in to the best research methodologies. Ethical issues, such as

> Consider whether the problems with the research were because of the researchers' error. It is often the case that a more perfect or more robust design and method would be fine in theory but impossible to conduct in practice.

the need to obtain informed consent and to ensure that participants are not harmed by the research, do often limit what can be done. It is the case, for example, that very little clinical research is undertaken on the use of drugs in babies and children. This is because it is often impossible to obtain their informed consent. In the same way, research that does take place in healthcare practice is often subject to design limitations. If you can show your understanding of these issues, rather than simply criticising the study for not being perfect, then you will have shown that you have a broad understanding of research issues.

Keep your essay simple. Research terminology is difficult enough to get to grips with, and the whole subject may be new to you. Keep it simple: do not be afraid to use language with which you are familiar rather than research language that you may not fully understand. If you make the mistake of using terminology with which you lack confidence, your lack of

> Keep it simple: do not be afraid to use language with which you are familiar rather than research language.

confidence will come across very clearly in your essay. Be content to use plain English and allow yourself to acclimatise to research terminology at your own pace.

Research ethics is an important subject. It may be that you have been asked specifically to write about ethics. However, unless you have been asked specifically to write about ethics, consider not allocating too much space to a critique of the ethics. The reason for this is that

> Unless you have been asked specifically to write about ethics, consider not allocating too much space to a critique of the ethics.

authors often don't have much space to discuss ethics within the limited word count that most journals specify. In practice, it is safe to assume that their research will have been processed by a properly appointed ethics committee. It is good to mention research ethics in your essay, but do not expect there to be a full account of the ethical issues in the research paper that you are critiquing.

Lastly, but importantly, be positive: show your enthusiasm for research. In healthcare practice, research and evidence-based practice are not yet perfect, but it is important to be able to

> Be positive: show your enthusiasm for healthcare and for research.

deal with the difficulties and have the enthusiasm and commitment to see how they can be improved. Remember: you are the future, and the examiner will want to see that you are enthusiastic about your profession.

You will meet practitioners whose only concerns are the here and nows of their present shift, their ward or area. There will probably be times when the here and now of busy practice will be your chief concern too. However, the professional practitioner also possesses a responsibility to the whole profession and to the care of patients in the future. Research is not without its difficulties, but it is a necessary endeavour for practice to progress and to improve. This book has been written to help students get both their feet firmly on the first two to three rungs of the ladder that is research. However, it isn't enough to understand research. At some point in your career you should become actively involved in research, so that you can play your part in the progress that your discipline must make to continue to provide patients with the care they need. Enjoy the challenge!

Appendix – Statistical Tests and Procedures

Analysis of variance (ANOVA)

A general term for a range of parametric statistical procedures designed to be run on interval and ratio data and which are generally used to identify the effect of one or more independent variables on one or more dependent variables in a manner that we would be likely to see in an experiment or clinical trial. Different forms of analysis of variance have been designed for different research designs. In this way, a 'one-way ANOVA' is used where there is one independent variable with 3 conditions (groups) and where there is one dependent variable.

Chi square (X²) (Pearson chi square)

Pearson chi square is used for nominal data (categories) where associations are hypothesised.

In this example, we can see an analysis run on fictitious data about males' and females' declared favourite colour. You can perhaps see that males are more likely to choose 'blue' and females are more likely to choose 'pink'. We can see that there is an association between the variables 'sex' and 'colour choice'. In other words, there is a difference between males and females in relation to their colour choice. We can also see, using Pearson Chi Square, that this result is significant, that it is unlikely to have occurred by chance.

Sex * Colour Crosstabulation

Count

		Colour		Total
		Pink	Blue	
Sex	Male	4	24	28
	Female	20	1	21
Total		24	25	49

Chi-Square Tests

	Value	df	Asymp. Sig. (2-sided)	Exact Sig. (2-sided)	Exact Sig. (1-sided)
Pearson Chi-Square	31.469[a]	1	.000		
Continuity Correction[b]	28.313	1	.000		
Likelihood Ratio	36.901	1	.000		
Fisher's Exact Test				.000	.000

Cronbach's alpha

Cronbach's alpha is used to test internal consistency or reliability. It is most commonly used to test that a questionnaire is 'reliable'. This is generally done by including questions in the questionnaire which ought to be answered in the same way as other questions.

Reliability Statistics

Cronbach's Alpha	N of Items
.971	8

Item-Total Statistics

	Scale Mean if Item Deleted	Scale Variance if Item Deleted	Corrected Item-Total Correlation	Cronbach's Alpha if Item Deleted
Italy	59.4907	31.201	.949	.963
South Korea	59.0810	31.513	.929	.964
Romania	59.8700	31.680	.934	.964
France	59.0210	33.146	.931	.966
China	59.9377	33.285	.942	.965
United States	59.1397	30.183	.924	.965
Russia	59.8230	30.273	.917	.965
Enthusiast	59.4713	32.666	.660	.981

In this example, the scores from eight judges were analysed to test for internal consistency (reliability, agreement). The Cronbach's alpha score is very high, indicating that there was a high level of agreement amongst the judges.

Friedman test

The Friedman test is a non-parametric equivalent of the one-way analysis of variance for a related design. The Friedman test can be run on ordinal data, or interval/ratio data which fails to meet the criteria for the use of a parametric test such as the one-way ANOVA.

The Freidman test is run where there is one variable which is measured on more than two occasions. For example, a physiotherapist tries to improve the evaluations of a patient fitness regime by getting each patient to undergo three fitness sessions in turn:

- The first one with rock music playing;
- The second session with country music playing;
- The third session with classical music playing.

The physiotherapist asks the patients to evaluate each session on a scale of 1 – 10.

The data look like this:

	Rock	Country	Classical	
0	1.00	4.00	7.00	
0	2.00	5.00	8.00	
0	3.00	6.00	9.00	
0	2.00	5.00	9.00	
0	1.00	4.00	7.00	
0	2.00	5.00	8.00	
0	2.00	6.00	8.00	
0	2.00	6.00	9.00	
0	1.00	5.00	8.00	
0	2.00	4.00	7.00	
0	1.00	4.00	8.00	
0	2.00	5.00	9.00	

And here are the results of the physio's analysis:

Descriptive Statistics

	N	Percentiles		
		25th	50th (Median)	75th
Rock music	64	2.0000	2.0000	3.0000
Country music	64	4.0000	5.0000	6.0000
Classical music	64	8.0000	8.0000	9.0000

Friedman Test

Ranks

	Mean Rank
Rock music	1.02
Country music	1.98
Classical music	3.00

Test Statistics[a]

N	64
Chi-Square	126.031
df	2
Asymp. Sig.	.000

a. Friedman Test

Because the data is ordinal, mean rank has been computed (instead of mean). We can see that the mean rank for classical music has the highest value. In the 'test statistics' box we can see (under Asymp. Sig) that the result is significant - so the three music groups do differ in a manner that would not have occurred by chance. We can see that the classical music group was evaluated best here. Sometimes, however, the result is less clear and we have to run 'post hoc' tests to determine which group is most different from the others.

Kruskal Wallis	The Kruskal Wallis test is a non-parametric equivalent of the one-way analysis of variance for unrelated groups. The Kruskal Wallis test can be run on ordinal data, or interval/ratio data which fails to meet the criteria for the use of a parametric test such as the one-way ANOVA.

For this statistical procedure, we would expect to have one independent variable with more than two conditions.

A doctor wants to test a new analgesic drug. However, a new form of intensive care is designed to enhance the effectiveness of the drug. Our doctor also wants to test the drug against a control group which would have no treatment (no drug and basic care only). So there are three conditions in the treatment variable:

(1) New drug

(2) New drug plus intensive care

(3) Control group.

The dependent variable is 'reported pain' which exists on a 1-10 scale.

Here is what the analysis looked like:

Kruskal–Wallis Test

Ranks

	Treatment	N	Mean Rank
Pain score (1–10)	1-New Drug	21	32.07
	2-New drug and special care	21	11.17
	3-Control	22	53.27
	Total	64	

Test Statistics[a,b]

	Pain score (1-10)
Chi-Square	55.949
df	2
Asymp. Sig.	.000

a. Kruskal Wallis Test
b. Grouping Variable: Treatment

We can see that there are quite large differences between the mean ranks for the three conditions. The new drug plus intensive care gets the lowest score, reflecting lower patient pain scores.

The analysis (Kruskal Wallis) shows a significant result, meaning that the groups are in fact different and to a degree that would not have occurred by chance.

The results seem pretty clear here. However, often it is necessary to run post hoc tests to clarify what exactly is the difference between the three groups.

Mann Whitney test

The Mann Whitney test is a non-parametric equivalent of the t-test for unrelated groups. The Mann Whitney test can be run on ordinal data or interval/ratio data which fails to meet the criteria for the use of a parametric test such as the t-test.

In a Mann Whitney test we would have one independent variable with two conditions. Let us say that we wish to test a new analgesic drug against a control. Our 'treatment' variable has two conditions:

- New drug

- Control

The dependent variable will consist of the patients' recorded pain levels, using a scale of 1-10.

Here are the test results:

Mann-Whitney Test

Ranks

	New drug versus control	N	Mean Rank	Sum of Ranks
Pain Scores - two conditions	(1) Control	33	47.94	1582.00
	(2) New Drug	31	16.06	498.00
	Total	64		

Test Statistics[a]

	Pain scores - two conditions
Mann-Whitney U	2.000
Wilcoxon W	498.000
Z	-6.926
Asymp. Sig. (2-tailed)	.000

a. Grouping Variable: New drug versus control

We can see that the mean rank for the control and for the new drug are quite different, with the new drug being associated with lower pain scores.

The result is significant (see the figure of .000 for Asymp Significance). This means that the difference we observe between the two groups is very unlikely to have occurred by chance.

Multivariate analysis of variance (MANOVA)

MANOVA is an extension of ANOVA and is principally different in that it can deal with more than one independent variable and more than one dependent variable. MANOVA is often used in psychology research and in other situations that are essentially 'multivariate'.

In multivariate analyses, the researcher will be aware that there are a number of variables interacting with each other and that it would therefore not be desirable to study each effect in isolation. Not surprisingly, multivariate analysis of variance can become very complicated.

In this analysis, we are seeking to find out whether field of practice (nurse, physio, etc) and sex (male, female) have an effect on the degree to which participants claim they like classroom study and practice experience. We also want to find out if there is an interaction between field of practice and the participant's sex in relation to their preference for practice experience or classroom study.

Here are the descriptive statistics (e.g. mean scores) for each field of practice, broken down in terms of participant sex.

Descriptive Statistics

	Field of Practice	Sex	Mean	Std. Deviation	N
Score for practice experience	(1) Nurse	Male	78.4000	15.22571	10
		Female	78.1429	11.11198	7
		Total	78.2941	13.29363	17
	(2) Physio	Male	73.7692	17.24410	13
		Female	78.0000	8.36660	5
		Total	74.9444	15.17146	18
	(3) Radiographer	Male	69.8182	12.97550	11
		Female	73.2857	12.27076	7
		Total	71.1667	12.45817	18
	(4) Medic	Female	79.7273	7.90052	11
		Total	79.7273	7.90052	11
	Total	Male	73.8529	15.29930	34
		Female	77.5667	9.70490	30
		Total	75.5938	13.01735	64
Score for classroom study	(1) Nurse	Male	41.6000	16.14655	10
		Female	32.1429	16.68761	7
		Total	37.7059	16.55583	17
	(2) Physio	Male	35.1538	16.84659	13
		Female	43.4000	19.03418	5
		Total	37.4444	17.32126	18
	(3) Radiographer	Male	44.2727	10.18912	11
		Female	34.7143	19.93083	7
		Total	40.5556	14.97536	18
	(4) Medic	Female	41.9091	16.10872	11
		Total	41.9091	16.10872	11
	Total	Male	40.0000	14.89560	34
		Female	38.2000	17.34717	30
		Total	39.1562	15.98632	64

From the above chart we are able to see that there is a clear preference for practice experience across all fields and across both sexes. However, there does not seem to be any difference between the scores for fields of practice and for sex.

Tests of Between-Subjects Effects

Source	Dependent Variable	Type III Sum of Squares	df	Mean Square	F	Sig.
Corrected Model	Score for practice experience	788.626[a]	6	131.438	.758	.606
	Score for classroom study	1211.769[b]	6	201.961	.773	.594
Intercept	Score for practice experience	359224.031	1	359224.031	2071.019	.000
	Score for classroom study	96979.735	1	96979.735	371.279	.000
Field	Score for practice experience	467.783	3	155.928	.899	.447
	Score for classroom study	261.409	3	87.136	.334	.801
Sex	Score for practice experience	73.480	1	73.480	.424	.518
	Score for classroom study	153.913	1	153.913	.589	.446
Field * Sex	Score for practice experience	46.046	2	23.023	.133	.876
	Score for classroom study	796.003	2	398.001	1.524	.227
Error	Score for practice experience	9886.812	57	173.453		
	Score for classroom study	14888.669	57	261.205		
Total	Score for practice experience	376398.000	64			
	Score for classroom study	114226.000	64			
Corrected Total	Score for practice experience	10675.438	63			
	Score for classroom study	16100.437	63			

a. R Squared = .074 (Adjusted R Squared = -.024)
b. R Squared = .075 (Adjusted R Squared = -.022)

The multivariate analysis of variance results are necessarily rather complex. However, if we look at the rows for field and sex and the interaction between field and sex, we can see that the results are non-significant. So, we can deduce that while all these people clearly prefer practice to study, there is no difference between them in terms of field of practice or their sex. It's quite simple; they all prefer practice to sitting in a classroom.

Normal distribution

Parametric statistical procedures usually require the data to be normally distributed. Non-parametric statistical procedures can work happily with data that is not normally distributed. If we want to run a parametric test, e.g. a t-test, on data, we should first check that the data is normally distributed. If we produce a frequency distribution of the data we should expect it to take the shape of a bell-shaped curve. Here is an example of data that does not quite do this. Here the date is skewed to the left:

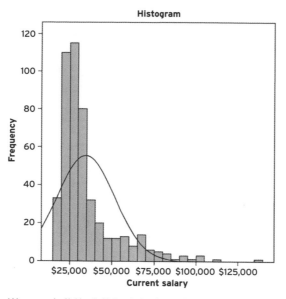

Histogram

We can tell that this data is not normally distributed, simply by looking at the graph. However, we can also run statistical tests on the data to give us an objective assessment of the distribution.

Tests of Normality

	Kolmogorov-Smirnov[a]			Shapiro-Wilk		
	Statistic	df	Sig.	Statistic	df	Sig.
Current Salary	.208	474	.000	.771	474	.000

a. Lilliefors Significance Correction

Here we see two tests which confirm our suspicion that this data is in fact not normally distributed. In circumstances like this one, we might choose to use non-parametric statistics or we might try to remove outlying values to try and normalise the data.

Normality tests (Kolmogorov-Smirnov test and Shapiro-Wilk test)

Let us say that a teacher wants to run a parametric statistical analysis on exam results data. The data are interval (a scale of 0-100). The data look like this:

Result
30.00
40.00
50.00
40.00
30.00
25.00
25.00
40.00
35.00
68.00
45.00
50.00
64.00
52.00

However, in order to be sure that the data meet the criteria for a parametric test, our teacher has to ensure that the data are normally distributed. So, she runs the Kolmogorov-Smirnov and Shapiro-Wilk tests (these two are run together in most statistical software packages). Here are the results:

Descriptives

			Statistic	Std. Error
Test Result	Mean		54.3281	2.24106
	95% Confidence Interval for Mean	Lower Bound	49.8497	
		Upper Bound	58.8065	
	5% Trimmed Mean		54.0694	
	Median		53.0000	
	Variance		321.430	
	Std. Deviation		17.92848	
	Minimum		12.00	
	Maximum		98.00	
	Range		86.00	
	Interquartile Range		21.75	
	Skewness		.316	.299
	Kurtosis		.000	.590

Tests of Normality

	Kolmogorov-Smirnov[a]			Shapiro-Wilk		
	Statistic	df	Sig.	Statistic	df	Sig.
Test Result	.089	64	.200[*]	.976	64	.259

a. Lilliefors Significance Correction
*. This is a lower bound of the true significance.

Along with some useful descriptive statistics for the data, we have results from the normality tests, both of which are non-significant, showing that the data are normally distributed.

So our teacher can now happily run her parametric tests on her data.

One-way ANOVA

This is used where differences are hypothesised and where there is one independent variable containing more than two conditions. The groups of data must be unrelated. One-way ANOVA is a parametric test and as such, the data must meet the criteria for a parametric design (see Parametric statistics). The Kruskal Wallis test is the non-parametric equivalent of the one-way ANOVA.

In this example, a drug at two separate dose levels are being used, along with a control group, to examine what effects it has on the blood levels of Seroptinine (fictitious). The independent variable has three conditions:

- Dose A
- Dose B
- Control group

The dependent variable is the recorded blood levels of Seroptinine.

Descriptive Statistics

Dependent Variable:Blood results

Treatment	Mean	Std. Deviation	N
1-Dose A	75.2381	16.06208	21
2-Dose B	76.2381	13.37126	21
3-Control	75.3182	9.57868	22
Total	75.5938	13.01735	64

Tests of Between-Subjects Effects

Dependent Variable:Blood results

Source	Type III Sum of Squares	df	Mean Square	F	Sig.
Corrected Model	13.046[a]	2	6.523	.037	.963
Intercept	365589.039	1	365589.039	2091.551	.000
Treatment3	13.046	2	6.523	.037	.963
Error	10662.392	61	174.793		
Total	376398.000	64			
Corrected Total	10675.438	63			

a. R Squared = .001 (Adjusted R Squared = -.032)

We can see that the mean values look much the same for the Dose A, B and control groups. It does not look at if either dosage has made any difference to the blood levels of Seroptinine. If we look at the analysis of variance table, we can see that the effect for 'Treatment3' is non-significant. So, it looks like we will have to try another dose!

One-way ANOVA (related)

This is used where differences are hypothesised and where there is one independent variable and where participants are exposed to the testing on more than two occasions. The design must be 'related' (e.g. the same participants are tested on more than two occasions). If testing takes place on only two occasions, a related t-test is used. One-way ANOVA is a parametric test and as such, the data must meet the criteria for a parametric design (see Parametric statistics). The non-parametric equivalent is the Friedman test.

In this example, we have males and females who undergo three patient education sessions. We wish to see if there is a difference between the males and females in terms of their knowledge at the end of each session (tested on a 1 – 100 scale).

Here are the descriptive statistics:

Descriptive Statistics

	Sex	Mean	Std. Deviation	N
Session One	Male	12.1471	6.76951	34
	Female	11.3333	5.74356	30
	Total	11.7656	6.27351	64
Session Two	Male	53.5588	5.77975	34
	Female	21.2333	5.25674	30
	Total	38.4062	17.16282	64
Session Three	Male	80.3824	8.57768	34
	Female	37.9000	5.61003	30
	Total	60.4688	22.57402	64

We can see that as the sessions progress, the male participants are increasing their knowledge (their score). However, the sessions do not seem to meet the needs of female participants; their score does increase but not by as much as does the score from the male participants.

Tests of Between-Subjects Effects

Measure:Class_scores
Transformed Variable:Average

Source	Type III Sum of Squares	df	Mean Square	F	Sig.
Intercept	249135.136	1	249135.136	8058.697	.000
Sex	30380.177	1	30380.177	982.698	.000
Error	1916.734	62	30.915		

If we now look at the test results for the one-way analysis of Variance (repeated measures), we can see that the effect for 'sex' is significant. This tells us that the difference in male and female scores which we see in the first table is unlikely to have occurred by chance. It looks like we will need to change the teaching sessions so that they better meet the needs of female participants.

Parametric statistics

Parametric statistics are a range of statistical procedures usually used on interval and ratio data. Examples of these procedures include t-test, ANOVA and MANOVA. These are some of the most useful and powerful statistical procedures available. However, to use these statistics, the data have to have the following characteristics (often called 'assumptions'):

- The dependent variable (e.g. recorded pain) is at the interval or ratio level of measurement;
- The dependent variable is approximately normally distributed;
- There is similar variance between the two groups (homogeneity of variance).

Fortunately, it is possibleto test the data to ensure these assumptions are met. It is also the case that many parametric statistical procedures can cope with data that do not quite meet the above criteria. Where there is concern, a non-parametric analysis may be chosen.

Paired samples t-test	See t-test (related).
Pearson chi square	See chi square.
Pearson rho (ρ)	The Pearson rho (rho is the Greek letter 'r') is a parametric correlation test. It is used to identify correlations between two variables where the data are at the interval or ratio level of measurement.

Let us use the example of children's age in months and their weight. These two variables should correlate because we know that, as children grow older, they tend to get heavier.

The data looks like this:

	Age	Weight
1	61.00	18.50
2	62.00	18.70
3	63.00	18.90
4	64.00	19.00
5	65.00	19.20
6	66.00	19.40
7	67.00	19.60
8	68.00	19.80
9	69.00	19.90
10	70.00	20.10
11	71.00	20.30

If we draw a scatter plot of the values and draw in a 'line of best fit', it will look like this (the values here are rather less scattered than one would expect in practice):

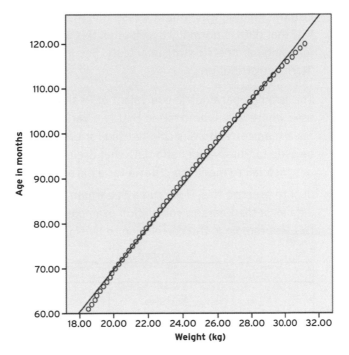

We can see that there is almost perfect correlation between age in months and weight.

Correlations

		Age in months	Weight (KG)
Age in months	Pearson Correlation	1	.999**
	Sig. (2-tailed)		.000
	N	60	60
Weight (KG)	Pearson Correlation	.999**	1
	Sig. (2-tailed)	.000	
	N	60	60

**. Correlation is significant at the 0.01 level (2-tailed).

The Pearson correlation result is (as we would expect) significant. This means that we can be reasonably sure that these results did not occur by chance.

Post hoc tests

Post hoc is Latin for 'after this'. Post hoc tests are run after analyses involving more than 2 conditions. This is because the main inferential statistics such as ANOVA will only tell us that there is a difference between the (3) groups, it will not tell us which group is most different from the other two. Examples of post hoc tests include Scheffé's and Tukey's tests.

Shapiro-Wilk test

Like the Kolmogorov-Smirnov test, the Shapiro-Wilk test is used to test that data is normally distributed, this being one of the criteria for using parametric statistical tests. See 'Normality tests' and 'Normal distribution'.

Spearman correlation

This is a non-parametric equivalent of Pearson's correlation. It is used where it is hypothesised that two variables are correlated. Spearman correlation is chiefly used for ordinal data but can also be used for interval or ratio data that are not normally distributed or which fail to meet the criteria for a parametric design.

Just to practise this, if we run a Spearman analysis on the same data as in the Pearson correlation example (above), we find that this test too, finds the correlation to be significant.

Correlations

			Age in months	Weight (KG)
Spearman's rho	Age in months	Correlation Coefficient	1.000	1.000**
		Sig. (2-tailed)	.	.
		N	60	60
	Weight (KG)	Correlation Coefficient	1.000**	1.000
		Sig. (2-tailed)	.	.
		N	60	60

**. Correlation is significant at the 0.01 level (2-tailed).

t-test

The t-test is a parametric test used to compare the effect of one independent variable (e.g. sex) with two conditions (e.g. male, female) on a dependent variable and where the design is unrelated. The data must be interval or ratio and must meet the criteria for a parametric design (see Parametric statistics). The non-parametric equivalent of the t-test is the Mann Whitney test.

Let us assume that we want to see if the blood levels of Seroptinine (fictitious) are different between males and females. In this case we have one independent variable (sex) with two conditions (male, female). The dependent variable is the blood levels of Seroptinine. Here are the results:

Group Statistics

	Sex	N	Mean	Std. Deviation	Std. Error Mean
Blood results	Male	34	73.8529	15.29930	2.62381
	Female	30	77.5667	9.70490	1.77186

We can see that the mean value for males and females is quite similar. When we run the t-test (below), we find that the result is not significant. So, there is no evidence here that males and females have different levels of Seroptinine.

Independent Samples Test

		Levene's Test for Equality of Variances		t-test for Equality of Means						
									95% Confidence Interval of the Difference	
		F	Sig.	t	df	Sig. (2-tailed)	Mean Difference	Std. Error Difference	Lower	Upper
Blood results	Equal variances assumed	8.881	.004	-1.142	62	.258	-3.71373	3.25289	-10.21616	2.78871
	Equal variances not assumed			-1.173	56.573	.246	-3.71373	3.16605	-10.05467	2.62722

t-test (related) or Paired samples t-test.	The t-test (related) is a parametric test used to compare the effect of the independent variable on the dependent variable as measured on two occasions. There must be two sets of data taken from the same participants (or matched participants) on two occasions. The data must be interval or ratio and must meet the criteria for a parametric design (see Parametric statistics). The non-parametric equivalent of this test is the Wilcoxon signed-rank test.

Let us take the example of blood cholesterol, taken from participants before and after a lifestyle-change programme designed to improve diet. A blood test is taken at the start of the programme and again, three months later. Here are the mean results (mmol/L).

Paired Samples Statistics

		Mean	N	Std. Deviation	Std. Error Mean
Pair 1	Start of programme	7.1267	30	.55890	.10204
	End of programme	3.7767	30	.51306	.09367

It certainly looks as if the programme has been successful. There has been a big drop in the mean cholesterol level. Now let's check to see if the result is statistically significant.

Paired Samples Test

		Paired Differences							
					95% Confidence Interval of the Difference				
		Mean	Std. Deviation	Std. Error Mean	Lower	Upper	t	df	Sig. (2-tailed)
Pair 1	Start of programme - End of programme	3.35000	.86053	.15711	3.02867	3.67133	21.322	29	.000

We can see from the above output that indeed, the result is significant (look at the box on the far right). This means that the difference we observed in the mean values is very unlikely to have occurred by chance but will have occurred as a result of the life-style change programme.

Two-way ANOVA	A two-way ANOVA is similar to a one-way ANOVA except that it can handle two independent variables. It is a parametric test and is used where there are two independent variables, each with one or more conditions (groups) and one dependent variable. If there is more than one dependent variable, a multivariate analysis of variance (MANOVA) should be used. There is essentially no non-parametric equivalent of the two-way ANOVA.

Wilcoxon signed-ranks test

The Wilcoxon signed-ranks test is a non-parametric equivalent of the related t-test. It is used where there is one independent variable with two conditions (groups) and where the design is related. In practice, there will be two sets of data taken on two occasions from either the same participants (on both of the two occasions) or from 'matched' participants.

Let's run the test on the same data we used for the paired samples t-test, assuming here that this data did not meet the criteria for a parametric design (for example, that the data are not normally distributed). This is data taken on two occasions and we are interested in seeing if there is a difference between the two sets of data – in this case that there is a reduction in serum cholesterol levels.

Here are the descriptive statistics. Again, there is a good indication (see the mean and median values) of a difference between the data obtained at the start of the programme and at the end of the programme.

Statistics

		Start of programme	End of programme
N	Valid	30	30
	Missing	0	0
Mean		7.1267	3.7767
Median		7.0500	3.6500

If we run the Wilcoxon signed-ranks test, we find, as expected, that the difference seen in the mean and median values for the two sets of data is statistically significant.

Test Statistics[b]

	End of programme - Start of programme
Z	-4.786[a]
Asymp. Sig. (2-tailed)	.000

a. Based on positive ranks.
b. Wilcoxon Signed Ranks Test

This means that we can expect that the change in blood cholesterol did not occur by chance.

Glossary of terms

Actor	A term used by ethnographers to mean 'research participant'.
Assumptions (data assumptions)	The criteria that data must meet in order for a test to be run on that data. For example, most parametric tests (e.g. ANOVA) require that:

- the dependent variable (e.g. recorded pain) is at the interval or ratio level of measurement;
- the dependent variable is approximately normally distributed;
- there is similar variance between the two groups (homogeneity of variance).

Statistical tests are available which can be run on the data to ensure that assumptions are met.

Audit trail	Clear documentation of each step in the research process – to enable a reviewer to trace each step – to make the research process transparent.
Axial coding	Identifying relationships between the identified categories (or themes) assigned to qualitative data.
Axiology	The study of values.
Between-group (difference, variance, effects)	The 'effect' (difference) found between (usually) the control group and the intervention group.

- Where the variance (difference) between the control and intervention groups is greater than the variation (difference) within each of the control and intervention groups, the result of the statistical procedure will tend to be significant.
- Where the variance within the control group and (separately) the intervention group is greater than the variance between the control and intervention groups, the result of the statistical test will tend to be non-significant.

Bias	The unwitting misrepresentation of data which causes the results to lack validity (be untrue). Bias is generally dealt with by blinding and by randomisation.

Bivariate

Involving two variables. Correlation studies tend to look at the degree to which one variable correlates with another variable (age and weight of children). Such studies are 'bivariate'.

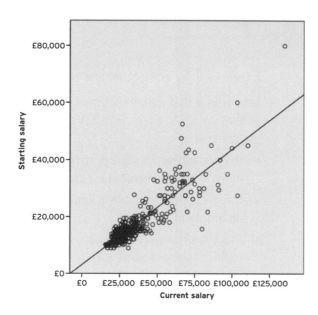

Chart showing the correlation of two variables: starting salary and current salary.

Blinding

Blinding is where the researcher and or the participant are unaware of whether they are in the intervention or the control group. Blinding is an important mechanism to reduce bias.

Categorical variable

A variable in the form of categories. Synonymous with 'nominal' data. For example:

Blue/red/pink/yellow;

Yes/no;

Correct/incorrect.

Conditions

Groups within an independent variable. For example, we may have the independent variable 'Treatment', which may contain two conditions: 'New drug' and 'Control' (no drug). This is one variable with two conditions.

Confidence interval

A confidence interval is a measure of how likely it is that a measure (e.g. the mean) taken from a sample would be found in the population. On the whole, long confidence intervals tend to be a bad thing, reducing our confidence that the sample is a valid representation of the population.

Descriptives

			Statistic	Std. Error
Current Salary	Mean		$34,419.57	$784.311
	95% Confidence Interval for Mean	Lower Bound	$32,878.40	
		Upper Bound	$35,960.73	
	5% Trimmed Mean		$32,455.19	
	Median		$28,875.00	
	Variance		2.916E8	
	Std. Deviation		$17,075.661	
	Minimum		$15,750	
	Maximum		$135,000	
	Range		$119,250	
	Interquartile Range		$13,163	
	Skewness		2.125	.112
	Kurtosis		5.378	.224

In this example, the confidence intervals give us an indication of how our measure (in this case, the mean salary) would be reflected in the population.

Confirmability	(Sometimes used in ethnography.) The degree to which it is possible to assess whether the findings flow from the data - i.e. is the study 'auditable'?
Constant comparative method	Where the researcher analyses the text on a continuous basis as new data is brought in, constantly examining and re-examining the text in relation to the developing themes or categories. This method is most closely associated with grounded theory but is often used in other forms of qualitative research.
Constructivist (interpretive) paradigm	The notion that much of the world is 'open to interpretation', that there is no objective truth or measurable facts and that instead, 'truth' is something that we perceive to be there. In this way, we all see things differently, and what is true for one person may not be true for another. Qualitative research largely accepts this interpretive approach.
Content analysis	An overarching term meaning any qualitative analysis. It Is interpreted by some as indicating a more descriptive (less interpretive) analysis.
Continuous data	Data existing as a scale or as ratio data with no end points to the scale (e.g. blood pressure, pulse rate). Synonymous with 'interval' and 'ratio' data, as in the 1-100 scale used by examiners when they mark students' essays.

The term 'continuous data' is used to differentiate the data from that obtained from (usually short) non-continuous scales such as the 5-point Likert scale. The Likert scale is not continuous because it is not possible to select '1.5' from the scale, even when that might be what we want to do (i.e. when it is meaningful).

Control, control group

The group to which the intervention being tested is **not** applied. The group to which the treatment (intervention) is applied is usually called the 'treatment group', or 'intervention group'. The control group allows for a comparison to be made with the treatment group. This comparison helps to determine that the effect caused has been due to the 'intervention' and that it would not have occurred without the intervention.

Correlation (correlational study)

The degree of interrelationship between two variables. The two variables – e.g. children's age in months and children's weight in kilograms – correlate positively. As children grow older, they tend to get heavier. In this case, each variable has a linear relationship to the other.

The fact that children's age and weight correlate does not mean that one variable causes the other, only that (in this case) they are linearly related (correlated). In most cases where correlation is used, the researcher will not be interested in determining causation. Thus, we would probably not be too interested in the notion that children's weight might cause their age.

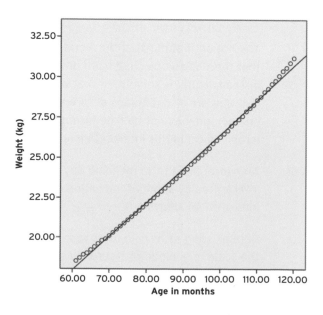

However, we are often interested in taking correlations further, because we are interested in determining whether one variable does have a causative impact on another variable. Regression procedures (such as linear regression) aim to determine whether one variable (the predictor variable) has an effect on the other variable (the dependent variable).

Credibility	Similar to internal validity. The degree to which the researcher's interpretation of the data can be justified in the data itself.
Data	Values or factual information collected during research. Note that 'data' is plural; the singular form is 'datum'.
Data saturation	The point at which new data from participants fails to add anything useful to the analysis. The data saturation point signals the completion of the data collection.
Deductive research	Research which starts with a hypothesis or is often carried out within a theoretical model, as in researching an aspect of Freudian theory. The researcher starts with preconceived ideas of what the data will be like. Common in psychological research.
Dependability	Similar to 'reliability'. If the study was repeated, similar results would be obtained.
Dependant variable	The variable that is being tested or acted upon by the independent variable. For example, in a randomised control trial, a new drug is given to one group of patients to see if it reduces reported pain levels. Treatment with the new drug is the independent variable and reported pain is the dependent variable. The independent variable (treatment) will probably have at least two subdivisions or 'conditions', these might, for example be 'New drug' and 'No drug' (control).
Descriptive statistics	Descriptive statistics describe the data, rather than drawing inferences from the data. Mean, mode and median are examples of descriptive statistics.
Descriptive study	The opposite of an experiment, a descriptive study seeks to describe what already exists. It is sometimes referred to as 'retrospective' (an experiment is 'prospective'). A survey is a good example of a descriptive study.

Design

The plan for the study. Well-known designs include 'pre-test-post-test' study and 'double-blind trial'. Design is often used with the word 'method', as in 'design and method'. 'Method' is the way the study will be carried out – for example, it might use questionnaires or a survey.

Differences

This is not an 'official' research term. However, it is often useful to differentiate correlational studies from those that are designed to demonstrate an effect of one variable upon another. In the latter case, we are usually looking at 'differences' or what changes an independent variable might make in a dependent variable.

Discourse analysis

The way language is used to represent social or cultural understanding of a phenomenon.

Discrete (data)

Data which exist as categories. Synonymous with 'nominal' or 'categorical' data.

Distribution (normal distribution)

Parametric statistical procedures usually require the data to be normally distributed. Non-parametric statistical procedures can work happily with data that is not normally distributed. If we want to run a parametric test (e.g. a t-test) on data, we should first check that the data is normally distributed. If we produce a frequency distribution of the data we should expect it to take the shape of a bell-shaped curve. Here is an example of data that does not quite do this. Here the data is skewed to the left:

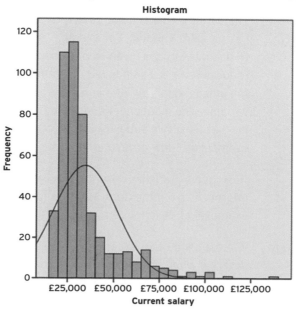

We can see that this data is not normally distributed, simply by looking at the graph. However, we can also run statistical tests on the data to give us an objective assessment of the distribution.

	Kolmogorov-Smirnov[a]			Shapiro-Wilk		
	Statistic	df	Sig.	Statistic	df	Sig.
Current Salary	.208	474	.000	.771	474	.000

Here we see two tests which confirm our suspicion that this data is, in fact, not normally distributed. In circumstances like this one, we might choose to use non-parametric statistics or we might try to remove outlying values to try and normalise the data.

Epistemology	The theory of knowledge (contrast with ontology – theory of meaning).
Ethnography	Ethnography is derived from anthropology and focuses on cultural meanings; how the organisation of society is achieved and the meaning people find in their culture or society.
Experiment	An experiment seeks to change something, that is, to cause an effect which can then be measured. An experiment is sometimes referred to as 'prospective' (a descriptive study may be described as 'retrospective').
Factor	A group or condition within an independent variable. Such groups are categorical. For example, an independent variable 'Treatment' might have two conditions, 'New drug' and 'Control'; in some forms of analysis, particularly ANOVA and MANOVA, these groups or conditions are known as 'factors'.
Framework analysis	A process of managing the coding of qualitative data and which involves the mapping of themes to cases.
Grounded theory	Focuses on generating theory on social processes by inductive examination of human experience. It is characterised by a close examination of the data together with reflection on the way it is being coded (constant comparative analysis). In practice, it is a relatively structured form of qualitative research which arguably comes closest to being a 'method'.

Groups   'Group' is a rather loose term which usually refers to a
                       condition or sometimes a dependent variable. A group will
                       always contain a set of data defined by a variable or by a
                       condition. Usually, 'group' means the same thing as 'condition'.

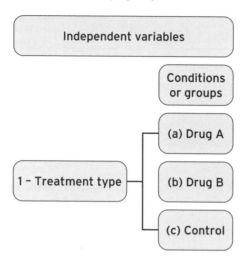

Hegemony   Imperial dominance. Sometimes used by qualitative
                       researchers to describe the dominance of quantitative
                       research (the hegemony of positivism).

Heideggerian   From Martin Heidegger (1889–1976), a German philosopher
hermeneutic   who further developed phenomenology from his one-time
phenomenology   teacher Husserl. Heideggerian phenomenology fully accepts
                       that truth can only be understood as a human or social
                       understanding (there is no objective reality). It contrasts with
                       Husserlian phenomenology, which argues that the qualitative
                       data remains essentially objective and measurable.

                       Heideggerian phenomenology accepts that the researcher is
                       an active participant in the research, where his or her own
                       experiences, values and beliefs are explicit.

Hermeneutic cycle   Philosophically, a system of interpretation that attempts to
(hermeneutics)   link unknown material to known meanings. In practice, it is
                       the Heideggerian notion that qualitative research should
                       legitimately be about interpretation of the participants'
                       experience. The researcher's interpretation of the data is
                       essentially subjective (though open to audit).

Husserlian phenomenology (Husserl's transcendental phenomenology)	After Edmund Husserl (1859–1938). Arguably, the first form of phenomenology which (like quantitative approaches) saw the researcher's experience, values and beliefs as a potential source of bias. In Husserlian phenomenology, the researcher tries to maintain a neutral position (known as 'bracketing') during the data collection and analysis. Usually contrasted with Heideggarian hermeneutic phenomenology.
Hypothesis	A statement of the expected outcome of the research, what 'effect' will be found. Traditionally, the hypothesis was expressed in negative terms, as a null hypothesis, which generally tended to state that an effect does **not** exist. In practice, a hypothesis is expressed as a way of stating exactly what the research is aiming to find out.
	It is not strictly necessary for a researcher to state the hypothesis. Many researchers are happy simply to identify the research question.
Independent variable	The 'treatment' variable. The variable introduced in an experiment to produce a change in the dependent variable. For example, in a randomised control trial, a new drug is given to one group of patients to see if it reduces their reported pain level. Treatment with the new drug is the independent variable and reported pain is the dependent variable. The independent variable (treatment) will probably have at least two sub-divisions or 'conditions', these might, for example be 'New drug' and 'No drug' (control).

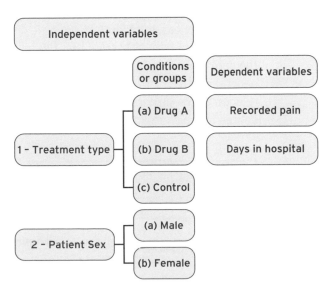

Inductive research	Research driven by questions about practice rather than theory. The researcher starts with an acknowledgement that little or nothing is known about the human experience in question.
Inferential statistics	Generally, those statistical procedures that are **not** descriptive statistics (such as mode, median, mean). Inferential statistics are so named because they draw inferences from the data. Inferential statistics are generally used to identify probability.
Interactionism	A term introduced by Herbert Blumer (1900–1987). A form of fieldwork which can be seen to form the basis of ethnography.
Interpretive paradigm	An acceptance that truth is subjective. Opposite of 'positivist paradigm'.
Interval data	A continuous scale (as in a 1–100 scale).
Intervention	The intervention is what is done to cause an effect. It is the effect of the independent variable on the dependent variable.
Likert scale	A scale of 1–5, usually dealt with using non-parametric statistical procedures (as with ordinal data). May sometimes be dealt with as categories (nominal).

I like Likert scales

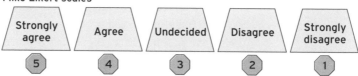

Mean (arithmetic mean)	A summary measure of interval and ratio data; the average value. It is important to bear in mind that the mean may not represent the data very well (the mean of 10, 10, 10, 10, 1, 1, 1, 1 is 5.5). In general, statistical procedures are interested in the mean in relation to the dispersion around the mean, the variance, the degree to which the mean does reflect the nature of the data.

Report

Test Result

Sex	Mean	N	Minimum	Maximum
Male	44.2059	34	12.00	68.00
Female	65.8000	30	32.00	98.00
Total	54.3281	64	12.00	98.00

Here is a report from a fictitious examination, showing the scores (marks) for males and females. The scale is 0–100. It looks as though the females performed better than the male students!

Median	Used as a summary measure of ordinal data. The median is the middle score of data placed in order of magnitude. The median of 12, 23, 34, 45, 56, 67, 78, 99, 100 is 56.

The median can be used with interval data to show whether the data is skewed (not normally distributed). Many statistical tests for interval/ratio data need the data to be normally distributed.

Statistics

Example ordinal data

N	Valid	64
	Missing	0
Median		3.0000

Example ordinal data

		Frequency	Percent	Valid Percent	Cumulative Percent
Valid	(1) Strongly disagree	11	17.2	17.2	17.2
	(2) Disagree	12	18.8	18.8	35.9
	(3) Not sure	17	26.6	26.6	62.5
	(4) Agree	12	18.8	18.8	81.3
	(5) Strongly agree	12	18.8	18.8	100.0
	Total	64	100.0	100.0	

Here is a frequency distribution taken from data derived from a Likert scale. We can see that the median value is 3 ('Not sure').

Member checking	The sharing of the summary or the analysis of the participant's data with the participant. Usually employed to achieve trustworthiness of the analysis.
Meta-analysis	An analysis run on data from more than one study. Meta-analyses are most commonly seen in systematic reviews where data from all the studies based on a particular clinical research question are amalgamated into one data set and analysed, usually by odds ratio or a similar statistical procedure.
Mixed methods	The use of two of more methods to access the same phenomenon. Often seen in triangulation studies. Can be a mix of different qualitative approaches or a mix of quantitative and qualitative approaches.
Mode	A summary measure of data. The mode is the most frequently occurring score in the set of data. It is most commonly used for categorical (nominal) data.

Statistics

Field of Practice

N	Valid	64
	Missing	0
Mode		2.00ᵃ

a. Multiple modes exist.
The smallest value is
shown

Field of Practice

		Frequency	Percent	Valid Percent	Cumulative Percent
Valid	(1) Nurse	17	26.6	26.6	26.6
	(2) Physio	18	28.1	28.1	54.7
	(3) Radiographer	18	28.1	28.1	82.8
	(4) Medic	11	17.2	17.2	100.0
	Total	64	100.0	100.0	

This is simply a frequency distribution of university healthcare students. The most frequently occurring value (mode) is '18', shared by physios and radiographers.

Multivariate	Involving many variables (or generally, more than two). It is generally better to isolate the one or two variables we wish to study than it is to pull lots of variables into the analysis. Research works better if it has a tight focus on just one phenomenon. However, human beings are essentially multivariate things and we are often aware that we cannot understand one variable without appreciating how that variable interacts with other variables. So it is that much of the research in psychology uses multivariate designs. It is important to understand that statistical procedures designed to work with several variables at once are designed to identify the 'interaction' between the variables. Such designs necessarily lead to some of the most complex statistical models.
Negative case analysis	A deliberate attempt to deal with aspects of the data which do **not** agree with the developing findings during the analysis of the data.
Nominal	Categories, such as (yes/no), (blue/white/red).
Non-parametric statistics	Non-parametric statistical procedures were mostly developed for ordinal data but they may also be used for interval and ratio data where they fail to meet the parametric criteria (assumptions).
	Non-parametric procedures (for example, the Mann-Whitney test) can be run on ordinal (non-continuous) data and where data is not normally distributed.

Odds ratio	The odds ratio is used in Cochrane Systematic Reviews. It is used in the meta-analysis of data combined from several or many studies. Risk ratio is a related statistic. See Chapter 6 for an example of the use of these statistics.
One-tailed/two-tailed (hypothesis, test)	The prediction of an effect in one direction only (one-tailed) or in either direction (two-tailed). Statistical procedures often provide a probability (significance) value for both one- and two-tailed analyses and it is up to the researcher to select the result that is most meaningful in relation to the hypothesis or research question. For example, we might hypothesise that the pain scores for those who received a new drug and those who did not (the control) would not just be different (two-tailed) but that the drug group would have the lower pain score (one-tailed).
Ontology	Theory of meaning. Contrast with 'epistemology' (theory of knowledge).
Open coding	Identifying categories (themes) in the data.
Ordinal data	Originally meaning data placed in order but generally meaning data in a short scale or a non-continuous scale, e.g. a 1–5 Likert scale. This is non-continuous because it is not possible to select 1.5, where 1.5 might be meaningful.
Parametric statistics	Parametric statistics are a range of statistical procedures usually used on interval and ratio data. Examples of these procedures include t-test, ANOVA and MANOVA. These are some of the most useful and powerful statistical procedures available. However, to use these statistics, the data has to have the following characteristics (often called 'assumptions'):

- The dependent variable (e.g. recorded pain) is at the interval or ratio level of measurement;
- The dependent variable is approximately normally distributed;
- There is similar variance between the two groups (homogeneity of variance).

Fortunately, it is possible to test the data to ensure these assumptions are met. It is also the case that many parametric statistical procedures can cope with data even if it doesn't quite meet the above criteria. Where there is concern, a non-parametric analysis may be chosen.

Peer de-briefing/ peer review	A process by which people not directly involved in the study are able to examine it. It is most usefully carried out when the study is being planned and during the course of the study.
Phenomenology	Experience of a phenomenon. In practice, phenomenology focuses on the interpretation of 'lived experience'.
Plausibility	The degree to which the researcher's interpretation of the data is likely to be realistic, given our existing knowledge.
Population	The potential data set to which the sample relates. When people are sampled to take part in a pre-election voting intention survey, the population is every eligible voter.
Positivist paradigm (positivism)	The notion that the world is chiefly an objective and measurable place. Positivism reflects our notion of science as it developed from the Reformation. Quantitative research largely accepts this positivist perspective. Opposite of 'interpretive paradigm'.
Post-modernism/ post-structuralism	A belief that there is no coherent way of explaining phenomena in structural terms. Tends to oppose the categorisation of phenomena or the use of structured research methods.
Post-test	The testing carried out after the 'treatment' (intervention).
Pragmatic paradigm	Where dealing with the research question is considered to be more important than adhering to a pure methodological approach.
Pre-test	The testing carried out before the 'treatment' (intervention).
Pre-test–post-test design	A study which in which testing takes place prior to the intervention and after the intervention – in order to determine the effect of the intervention. A control group may also be used which helps to determine whether any effect may have been due to the passage of time or to engagement between the researcher and the patient.
Probability (P-value)	Almost all inferential statistics exist to identify probability. We need to understand that 'chance' is everywhere in science. Chance is the part of the universe or of the research study that we do not understand, cannot anticipate and may not even know exists. Whenever we try to demonstrate that one variable has an effect on another variable or that two variables are correlated, we need to be able to show what 'risk' there is that the result we have obtained was caused only by chance.

Probability gives us a numerical figure for that risk. This is usually expressed as P=something. P=0.05 means that there is a 5% risk that the result was due to chance. P=0.01 means that there is a 1% risk.

Probability does not indicate the size of the effect but how sure we are that the effect we see was not caused by chance.

The word 'significant' is used when we are satisfied that the probability of the effect being caused only by chance is too small to worry about. However, there is no absolute value for significance. A 5% risk that the result may be due to chance may satisfy one person but not another person. It is arguably the case that research into treatments that are dangerous and life-threatening will (and should) be expected to achieve higher levels of significance than is the case in other forms of research.

| Prolonged engagement | An aspect of the quality of research (trustworthiness). The longer the time the researcher spends with participants, the richer and more understood will be the data and the interpretation of it. |

| Q-Q plot | The Q-Q plot is a graphical illustration of the degree to which data is normally distributed. Data needs to be normally distributed if parametric tests such as the t-test are to be used. |

This chart shows a Q-Q plot from data that is not normally distributed. For the data to be normally distributed we would expect to see the plots close to the diagonal line.

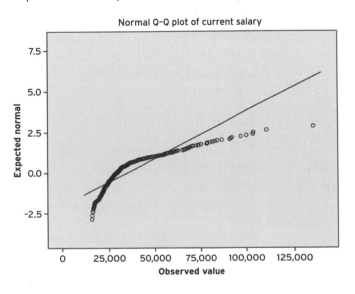

Normal Q-Q plot of current salary

Qualitative research

Qualitative research generally deals with spoken or written language. It usually starts with a question like 'How do people experience this particular health problem?' and explores a phenomenon from a starting position that is assumed to be one of ignorance. The starting point is the question itself, not a theory or an assumed knowledge base (it is 'inductive'). Qualitative research is used when we know so little about a human experience that we do not know exactly what questions to ask. Instead we use prompts such as 'Tell me what you felt about being in hospital.'

Quantitative research

This is research that we most clearly associate with traditional science. Quantitative research usually deals with numbers rather than text and, as the term suggests, deals with the 'quantity' of something. For example, we might measure patients' anxiety by asking them to allocate a number from 1 to 5 to indicate how anxious they are.

Radical (critical) interpretivism

A form of phenomenology which seeks not merely to describe experiences but to change them. Most clearly seen in research on feminism and social justice.

Randomisation

A process of recruiting participants or allocating participants to groups, where potential participants have an equal chance of being selected. Randomisation, together with 'control' (groups which do not have the treatment), is a central aspect of randomised control trials. Randomisation is considered an important mechanism by which a study may be judged to be robust, or of good quality. However, randomisation in some circumstances is difficult or impossible to achieve. This is especially true in healthcare research, where the random allocation of an individual to a treatment or control group may be unethical.

Randomised control trial (RCT)

An experiment (a prospective study) which includes randomisation, a control group and (usually) blinding.

Ranked data (ranking)

Data that is put in order (as in 12, 23, 45, 67, 99) or that already exists as ordered data. Ranked (ordered, ordinal) data is generally analysed by non-parametric statistical tests.

Ratio data

A continuous scale with no end points (e.g. blood pressure, serum cholesterol). In practice, interval and ratio data are treated much the same in statistical analyses.

Raw data   Data before they are analysed - the actual stuff collected by researchers.

Realism   Belief in a stable and objective reality.

Recruitment   The process of including participants in a qualitative study. In quantitative studies, the word 'sampling' is used.

Reflexivity   Researcher self-scrutiny - examination of the researcher's role in the research. Almost identical to the 'reflective practice' seen in healthcare today.

Regression   Regression procedures (such as linear regression) aim to
analysis   determine whether one variable (the predictor variable) has an effect on another variable (the dependent variable). Regression analysis was originally developed as an extension of correlational analysis. These days, forms of regression analysis are available for nominal, ordinal and interval data and for situations where a linear relationship between the two variables is not expected.

Related design   A related design is one where the same individuals (or matched, paired individuals) are tested on more than on occasion.

                    For example, a study may want to test the effect of a patient education programme on the advantages of adhering to diet in diabetes. The study is interested in how patients' attitudes to diet-adherence change over the time the programme is running (and perhaps afterwards). In order to achieve this, each participant has a diet-adherence attitude test each month for 6 months.

                    An unrelated design is one in which one group of participants is compared to another (separate) group of participants, in order to identify differences between the two groups.

Relativism   Belief in a socially constructed reality.

Reliability   The degree to which the same results would be obtained if the study were to be repeated.

                    Reliability can relate to data collection instruments. For example, a questionnaire might contain two questions which 'ought' to have the same answer. The degree of agreement between the two questions can be tested by using statistics designed to measure reliability.

Rigour	The quality of research, how capably it is done. 'Rigour' is a quantitative term and is usually substituted by 'trustworthiness' in qualitative research.
Robust	A general term describing the quality of a research study.
Sample	The part of the population of cases (all possible cases) that is used within the research study. For example, we might want to measure the quality of hand-washing in orthopaedic wards. Instead of looking at every orthopaedic ward in the world, we sample three orthopaedic wards in the UK and collect data on hand-washing just from those three wards. A sample should be representative of the population, although the researcher is often free to define the population (as just UK orthopaedic wards, for example).
Sampling	The procedure (method) used to produce the sample.
Scale	Any data that are distributed between two points; they may be either ordinal or interval. Statisticians tend to use the word 'scale' to mean interval or ratio data (as in 'continuous scale').
Selective coding	The process of identifying the core or central category (theme) from those identified during the analysis of qualitative data. All or most of the other categories will link with the main category. Used in grounded theory.
Significance (level)	Probability.
Standard deviation	Standard deviation is a measure of dispersion around the mean, or the within-group variability. A large standard deviation tends not be a good thing. If data for one variable varies a lot, it may indicate that there are problems with the data; it will also increase the likelihood that an analysis using that variable will return a non-significant result.
	Let's look at a data set containing pain scores from patients who received a new analgesic drug. Here are the descriptive statistics:

Descriptives

			Statistic	Std. Error
Standard Deviation	Mean		4.4688	.43414
	95% Confidence Interval for Mean	Lower Bound	3.6012	
		Upper Bound	5.3363	
	5% Trimmed Mean		4.3750	
	Median		2.0000	
	Variance		12.063	
	Std. Deviation		3.47311	
	Minimum		1.00	
	Maximum		10.00	
	Range		9.00	
	Interquartile Range		6.00	
	Skewness		.391	.299
	Kurtosis		-1.778	.590

We can see that the mean for the data on this 1–10 scale is 4.4688. We might assume that this figure usefully summarises our data. We might think that 'most' patients score around 4.5. However, if we look at the standard deviation, we see that it is quite large (3.47). This should alert us to the fact that something might be wrong with our data. Let's just take a closer look at actual scores:

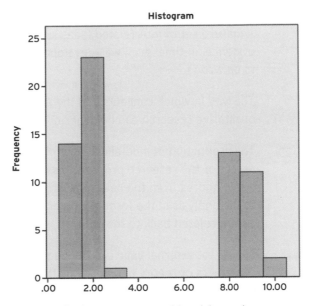

Histogram

Oops! In fact, our mean could not have done a worse job at summarising this data; none of the data are anywhere near the mean.

Survey	A descriptive study (not an experiment) generally having just one 'group'.

Survival analysis	A range of statistical procedures, including the Kaplan-Meier survival procedure, designed to identify the impact of an independent variable on 'survival'. The survival variable is time. In medical research, survival analysis is well-named because such research does often look at the impact of a new drug on the length of time to patient death. However, survival analysis can look at the impact of an independent variable on any dependent variable that is measured in time (such as the length of time nurses stay in clinical practice).
Systematic review (Cochrane systematic review)	Systematic reviews generally involve a meta-analysis of research data from several studies. The process is able to deal statistically with the issue of conflicting results from a number of studies focused on one clinical issue. See Chapter 6 for more information on systematic reviews.
Text	Sometimes used by qualitative researchers, meaning 'data'.
Thematic analysis	The development of themes in qualitative analysis. A theme is a word or construct which represents part of the data. The words 'code' and 'category' have a similar meaning.
Theory	A mature set of interrelated ideas supported by at least some evidence. In time, even well-developed theory may be shown to be wrong.
Theoretical generalisability	The way in which concepts and theories derived from qualitative research can be generalised.
Thick description	The production of a detailed description of the data and each aspect of the research process. Researchers will often use direct quotes from the data to illustrate how the conclusions to the analysis in the form of concepts, constructs or theory can be related back to the data.
Transferability	Similar to 'external validity'. The degree to which the concepts, constructs or theory generated by the analysis can be applied elsewhere.
Triangulation	A technique where more than one method is used to collect data on one phenomenon (method triangulation) or to analyse data (analysis triangulation). Can be used to enhance the credibility or trustworthiness of a study or to access a more complete understanding of the phenomenon.

Trustworthiness	The quality of research, how capably it is done. 'Trustworthiness' is the qualitative equivalent of the term 'rigour' used in quantitative research.
Univariate	Involving only one variable. A univariate analysis is an analysis run on just one variable. Descriptive statistics, such as mean and mode are univariate statistics.
Unrelated (unrelated design)	Data is collected from two or more separate groups of participants where differences between the groups are hypothesised.
Validity	Literally 'truth'. There are generally considered to be two forms of validity:

- Internal validity: the degree to which the researcher's interpretation of the data can be justified from the data itself. The degree to which the data is what we think it is (that it is true or 'valid');

- External validity: the degree to which the results of the study can be generalised to the relevant population.

Variable	Literally, something that varies. In practice, a variable is either the 'thing' that we are measuring (usually the dependant variable) or the 'thing' that we think will cause an effect on what we are interested in measuring (the independent variable).

Variable is a good name for these 'things' because it is the degree to which the data they represent vary within variables (within-group variability) and the degree of variation between variables (between-group variability) that is measured by most inferential statistical procedures. Variability is almost the bread and butter of statistics.

We might consider variability as 'change'. So, when we look at whether a new drug is impacting on reported pain levels, we are looking to see if the new drug 'changes' the reported pain levels.

If the variability between the treatment and control groups is great, and the variability within each set of data for the treatment and control groups (separately) is small, then we will tend to see the result returned as significant.

The standard deviation is generally used to measure the variation within a variable.

Within-group (difference, variance, effects)

The amount of variation (difference) that exists within one variable.

- Where the variance (difference) between the control and intervention groups is greater than the variation (difference) within each of the control and intervention groups, the result of the statistical procedure will tend to be significant.

- Where the variance within the control group and (separately) the intervention group is greater than the variance between the control and intervention groups, the result of the statistical test will tend to be non-significant.

Index

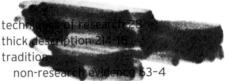

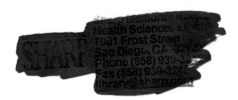